Tired of Being Tired

Rescue · Repair · Rejuvenate

Tired of Being Tired

JESSE LYNN HANLEY, M.D.,
and
NANCY DEVILLE

G. P. PUTNAM'S SONS
New York

Every effort has been made to ensure that the information contained in this book is complete and accurate. However, neither the publisher nor the author is engaged in rendering professional advice or services to the individual reader. The ideas, procedures, and suggestions contained in this book are not intended as a substitute for consulting with your physician. All matters regarding your health require medical supervision. Neither the author nor the publisher shall be liable or responsible for any loss or damage allegedly arising from any information or suggestion in this book.

The recipes contained in this book are to be followed exactly as written. Neither the publisher nor the author is responsible for your specific health or allergy needs that may require medical supervision, or for any adverse reactions to the recipes contained in this book.

G. P. Putnam's Sons
Publishers Since 1838
a member of
Penguin Putnam Inc.
375 Hudson Street
New York, NY 10014

Library of Congress Cataloging-in-Publication Data

Hanley, Jesse.
Tired of being tired : rescue, repair, rejuvenate /
Jesse Lynn Hanley and Nancy Deville.
p.   cm.
Includes bibliographical references and index.
ISBN 0-399-14749-7
1. Longevity.   2. Aging—Prevention.   3. Vitality.   4. Health.
I. Deville, Nancy.   II. Title.

RA776.75.H36   2001   00-066475
613—dc21

Printed in the United States of America

1   3   5   7   9   10   8   6   4   2

This book is printed on acid-free paper. ∞

Book design by Lee Fukui

Acknowledgments

This book began with a casual conversation with our agent, Ling Lucas, about the epidemic of adrenal burnout. Ling refused to let the idea go and deserves our first thanks, because without her inspiration this book would not have been written. Her driving force, encouragement, and guidance carried us through from the conceptual phase through the writing and editorial process.

We are most grateful to Phyllis Grann and Susan Petersen Kennedy at Putnam for their enthusiasm and support for this subject. Amy Hertz, our editor at Putnam, was a pleasure to work with. Her professionalism and expertise made this a more accessible and useful book. Amy's assistant, Rebecca Thomas, organized loose ends and kept us coordinated. Thanks also to copyeditors Martha Ramsey and Timothy Meyer, who did a wonderful job.

Early on in the writing, Dr. John A. Davis volunteered to read and edit our drafts, a task that stretched over many months. His careful reading, insightful comments, and suggestions helped shape many of the chapters.

Those who shared their real-life stories of adrenal burnout are the essence of this book, which would not have been nearly as readable and insightful without their contributions.

A task like this cannot be accomplished without a significant research support system. Ours included De'in Sofley, who painstakingly researched medical journals, transcribed hundreds of hours of tapes, and cheerfully took care of endless details. Others who brought order and organization to the process were David Stanley, Renée Perez, Courtney Sampson, Martha Dominguez-Smith, and Jennifer Thompson.

The scientists, doctors, health care professionals, and fitness authorities who lent their expertise to the research and writing of this book put the meat on the bones of many of the subjects: Aristo Wojdani, Ph.D., director of the Immunosciences Laboratory; David Steinman, nationally recognized authority on environmental toxins; Don Campbell, author and lecturer on the Mozart Effect; Erich Schiffmann, author, lecturer, and yoga master; Glenn Miller, M.D., physician, psychiatrist, and pharmacist; Josette Troxler, M.P.T., yoga therapist; Mary Enig, Ph.D., author and internationally recognized biochemist in the field of fats and oils and authority on transfatty acids; Dr. Peter Kulish, author and senior research scientist of the Magnetizer Biomagnetic Research Institute; Robert Becker, M.D., author and internationally recognized authority on electropollution; Robin Marzi, R.D., nutritional authority and William Philpott, M.D., author, neurologist, psychiatrist, and allergist.

We also thank Lyra Heller for championing the formulation of quality products for the treatment of adrenal burnout.

Over the past twenty years a number of doctors and scientists have helped shape Dr. Hanley's expertise; among them are Murray Susser, M.D., Hyla Cass, M.D., Cynthia Watson, M.D., Alan Green, M.D., Melvyn Werbach, M.D., Michael Rosenbaum, M.D., Jim Blechman, M.D., Janet Zand, N.D., Marcus Laux, N.D., and Michael Borkin, N.D. In addition, Jeffrey Bland, Ph.D., whose life's work has been dedicated to integrating nutritional/genetic biochemistry into the field of functional medicine, and Tom Newmark, president of New Chapter Vitamins, who introduced Dr. Hanley to holy basil. Profound gratitude from Dr. Hanley to her sister Pamela Serure, whose unending support, patience, and humor helped make this creative process a breeze.

Heartfelt gratitude from Nancy Deville to Stella Grabowski, Evelyn Jacob Jaffe, Grace Gabe, M.D., Cathy Quinn, Ph.D., and Susan Jenks Dudley Wigglesworth.

This book is dedicated to the loving memory of my mother, who taught me the most important lesson in life—love heals, starting with loving yourself.

—JLH

To John

—ND

Contents

Part Three
Eat Regular Balanced Meals of Real
Whole Food to Take Back Your Life

Tired of Being Tired

Introduction

At forty-three, Jessica Inman was overweight, tired, stressed out, and having stomach pains.* She was uninspired by her career. "Food had become a constant companion," Jessica said. "I was in a pattern of gaining and losing ten or fifteen pounds." Between the stress of family and career there never seemed to be enough time to think about making changes. Does Jessica's story sound familiar?

Maybe, like Jessica, your life is complete on the outside but empty on the inside. Has success brought you rewards, but have you no energy to enjoy them? Are you exhausted, struggling with health issues, and futilely battling your weight? Do you find you just do not have the vitality and optimism you once had? Do you suffer from insomnia and obsessive thoughts? Does it take one, two, three, or more cups of coffee just to get through the morning? You may think, I am getting older and this is what happens. It may be a surprise to learn that these symptoms are not a function of age. You do not have to slide into a helpless pattern of fatigue, weight gain—and illness. You can have your energy back, lose weight, sleep soundly, achieve optimal health, and look and feel younger.

When Jessica was offered a few simple solutions, she felt hopeful again. Within one month of making a few changes to her diet and taking the right supplements she began to feel better. Within two

---

* The people in this book and their stories are true. Some of their names and identifying characteristics and facts have been changed to protect their privacy.

1

months she had lost weight and had much more energy. "I wasn't really prepared for how good I would feel," Jessica said. "I started to get excited about my new business and getting my life back together. I have so many things going on that feeling healthy and balanced gives me an incredible foundation. I think that the more that you can be at your peak performance, the more you can give back to the lives of other people. And the more active you can be, the better you feel about yourself. Now that I've made some changes and have gotten such great results I'm really focused on changing other habits and I feel motivated."

Like Jessica, I am grateful for the health problems that I had early in life because they led me to make even more changes—which led me to where I am today. When I was growing up my mother gave me sugared and processed cereal for breakfast, hot dogs on white flour buns with pickles, and a Coke for lunch, and TV dinners—exactly what television in the 1950s suggested a good mother should feed her child. My parents were smokers, so I grew up in a smoke-filled home. I was chronically sick with tonsillitis and stomach problems, and I caught every infection that was going around. Antibiotics were such a regular part of my life then that I took them the way I take vitamins today. I was always so tired that I would often come home from school and fall asleep on my bed. I had no idea that sugar, secondhand smoke, processed foods, and even the antibiotics were causing my fatigue and health problems. In fact, in my teenage years I thought it was cool that I lived from candy bar to candy bar, not realizing that I was really starving my body.

One morning at age seventeen, while washing my face at the bathroom sink, I caught my exhausted reflection in the mirror and instantly realized that I was sick and tired of being sick and tired. I knew I had to do something about it. On the way home from school that day I passed by a neighborhood health food store, something I had done every day for years. That day I went inside and met a man who gave me my first lessons in natural health. What he said made such an impression on me that I began to read everything I could get my hands on about health and healing. I learned how to prepare whole foods and about the nutrients I needed. Four years later I realized that it had been four years since I had been sick.

Just as that wise man had helped me, it became my passion to help others be healthy. I cooked for them, helped them quit smoking, and did for them whatever was within my budding repertoire of healing. My passion led me to the Abraham Lincoln School of Medicine at the University of Illinois. I wanted to teach what I experienced—that health, energy, and vitality are a choice. I studied biochemistry, physiology, and endocrinology; simultaneously, I studied Oriental medicine at the UCLA Medical School, where I learned about Chinese herbal medicine and acupuncture. I also studied polarity therapy, which, like Chinese medicine, understands the body as an interconnected system of flowing energy. I found I could use alternative natural methods—such as nutrition, supplements, and lifestyle changes—to help people heal. Over the last twenty-five years I have successfully assisted thousands of people in their recovery from illnesses by using natural methods.

When I became the medical director of the Malibu Health Center in 1988, my practice filled up with extremely driven and stressed-out people. Every day people come into my office asking why they are overweight, anxious, and depressed; why they suffer from obsessive thoughts; why they are exhausted but cannot sleep; why they helplessly crave junk food and sugar; why it takes a pot of coffee to keep them going. Over the past twenty-five years I have witnessed miracles in the lives of these very same people. It all began with a few simple changes.

On a daily basis I hear people say they believe it is difficult to make changes. That is why my emphasis is on making small changes that make huge differences. More important, small changes make it easier for you to see that further changes are possible. The Ten Simple Solutions you will learn about in later chapters are designed to renew your energy, eliminate insomnia, reverse accelerated aging, help you look and feel younger, lose weight, restore immunity, and prevent illness.

This book was written because I know that people feel their lives are out of control and that there is nothing they can do to feel better. The truth is that you can have your energy back, lose weight, sleep soundly, and more. You can take your life back. I have seen it happen for many, and I would like to show you how to do it yourself. It is as easy as Ten Simple Solutions.

Part One

The Psychology and
Physiology of Highly
Ambitious People

The Adrenaline
Rush Lifestyle

It is habit forming

Nineteen-year-old Jenny Harrington, known to her friends as "Scout," lives with eight other coeds in a house near the beach close to the university they attend. She has lived there now for three summer months, and while the party animals play in the surf every day, Scout has yet to go to the beach once. To the other girls in her house Scout is a phantom who comes and goes with rarely a sighting.

Scout is in the early stages of success, which of course begins with ambition. At fifteen, she got her first job at a hot dog stand in the local mall. She was quickly promoted to assistant manager and was transferred to another store close to her college. In her freshman year, Scout took four classes each quarter in addition to working a forty-hour week, sleeping no more than five hours a night.

Highly ambitious people tend to love the adrenaline rush, risk-taking, and rising to challenges. At nineteen years old, Scout's duties at work include interviewing, hiring, and training and firing employees as well as approving raises, promotions, and demotions, ordering stock, repairing and maintaining the store, and riding herd on her crew's morale. She often works overtime, without pay, to accomplish her tasks. "Being a new manager, I get the nervous jitters when I have to face a new challenge like talking to the CEO or payroll people or employees," Scout said. "Every once in a while, I'm not sure if I know exactly how to handle things. But every time I'm successful I'm so excited. It's what keeps me thinking I'm going in the right direction." Financially, Scout is on her own. She attends college on a full scholarship, has recently bought a new car, and covers all of her own expenses.

Scout's story may provoke fond memories of the way it used to be for you. You used to be idealistic and ambitious too. Unfortunately, as people progress along in life, they often become more and more successful but less able to enjoy the fruits of their labors. You have it all, but you feel too tired or too overscheduled to enjoy what you have earned. It is just not as much fun as it used to be. You may wonder how it happened. You may feel that there is nothing you can do about it now; that it is too late. There is actually plenty you can do about it. You can feel better, look better, be healthier, sleep more soundly, and so much more.

Before I discuss how that can happen, let's flash forward from where Scout is to twenty-five years later so you can understand how you progressed to where you are today.

Fifty-two-year-old Rachel Kantor is a petite blonde who has been caught in the adrenaline rush lifestyle for many years. At one time, Rachel had over one hundred people working in her commercial real estate research and consulting firm, which she described as a "competitive, deadline business." She tightly choreographed the work because it "all had to come together brilliantly with no mistakes and exactly at the right time." Rachel, who describes herself as a "deadline person," did not recognize or care about the intense stress she was under. She worked all-nighters whenever a job required her to do so. She ran on empty, preferring the high she got from hunger to the "full sleepy feeling" she got from eating. "There's an adrenaline thing going on when you are not eating and you are working hard and feeling edgy," she said. "I love being on the edge with that feeling of everything being sharp. It's almost like taking uppers and having a high." Indeed, the adrenaline rush is very much like the high you get from drugs. And it just so happens that the adrenaline rush is the high that seduces many people.

Stress hormones such as adrenaline are secreted from your adrenal glands to prepare the body for acute and chronic physical and emotional stress. Most of us have heard of the adrenal glands, but very few people understand how they function and why they are important. Your two adrenal glands are triangular-shaped organs weighing less than five grams each that rest one above each kidney. These glands—about the size of two or three pinto beans each—secrete adrenaline and other stress hormones that influence nearly every bodily function.

The release of adrenaline is roughly proportional to the intensity of a situation. In other words, the amount of stress hormones that are secreted, and at what intervals, is determined by the degree of "danger" perceived by the brain. Encountering a great white shark while on vacation would elicit a larger and longer adrenaline response than going to a surprise birthday party in your honor. The adrenaline response occurs in the time it takes to snap your fingers.

The neo-cortex of the brain supposedly differentiates humans from all other animals. It is where memory, learning, speaking, and other intellectual functions, including processing the stimuli from your world, take place. The neo-cortex initially registers any given experience. Beneath the neo-cortex is the limbic system, which is sometimes referred to as the emotional brain. The limbic system translates sensory input into emotion. Instantaneously, your hypothalamus registers this information. Simultaneously, the sympathetic mode of your autonomic nervous system reacts, causing the rapid release of adrenaline, the fight-or-flight hormone from your adrenal medulla—the inner portion of your adrenal glands.*

---

* Hans Selye, internationally acknowledged as the father of the stress field, coined the term "fight-or-flight." After publishing the first scientific paper to identify and define "stress" in 1936, Selye wrote over seventeen hundred scholarly papers as well as thirty-nine books on the subject.

The adrenal medulla synthesizes, stores, and releases epinephrine and norepinephrine. For simplicity's sake, I will refer to these two hormones as adrenaline.

The adrenaline response can also be secreted without an emotional trigger. You could be in a serious car accident and be unconscious, and your adrenals would be pumping adrenaline like crazy in an attempt to manage your blood pressure and to otherwise stabilize your body in a life-threatening situation.

Although fear and danger are the greatest motivators of the adrenaline response, *all* of your excitatory experiences result in what Rachel referred to as a rush. In other words, experiences that are stimulating, such as getting an unexpected bonus at work, result in this high. Nonstimulating experiences, such as vegging out in front of the TV or ironing, generally do not. The sensation of the adrenaline rush is caused by the release of three factors into your system at the same time: (1) energy from sugar stored in your liver and muscles; (2) the feel-good neurotransmitter dopamine; and (3) internally created opiates called endorphins. With the release of these three factors you suddenly feel energized, fully alert, and euphoric.

The adrenaline response dates back tens of thousands of years to when the fight-or-flight response meant the difference between a prehistoric human's life or death. This survival reaction was appropriate thousands of years ago because it was a response to *dramatic danger*—like being chased by a wild animal that was intent on eating you. Today, this adrenaline response is rarely appropriate, but it is hardwired in us. Whether you get out of bed and stumble over your cat in the middle of the night, become engaged to be married, close a major deal at work, or hear your checkbook bouncing, you will experience some degree of the same adrenaline-related reaction as did our ancestors living in the wild.

We live in exciting times. Opportunity is exploding exponentially. We are like kids in a candy store, not wanting to miss out on a waking moment. A highly ambitious, successful forty-three-year-old physician/entrepreneur explained his philosophy by quoting the old adage: "I would rather crash and burn than rust away." A thirty-year-old restauranteur has spent three years developing a new dining concept—a feat that has required many twenty-hour days and virtually no weekends off. "I don't want my headstone to be blank," he explained. "I want my life to be a good story and that is really the driving factor.

Figure 1
Adrenaline response

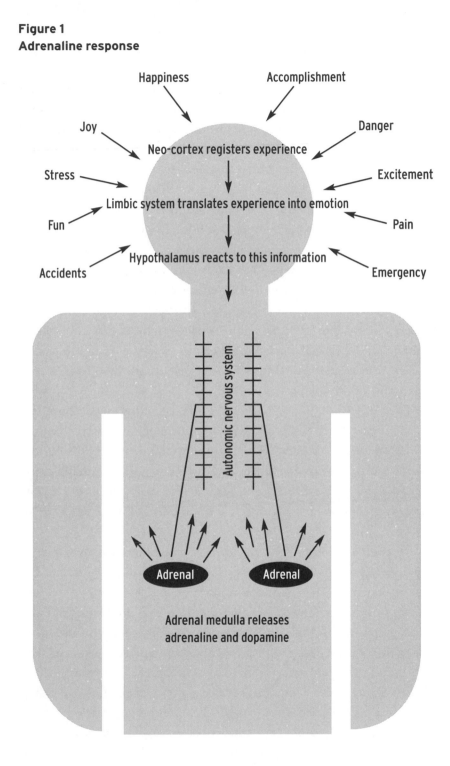

I want to feel that I have accomplished something." Both of these people, while working crazy hours and putting themselves under a lot of stress, feel that the effort has been worth it—and that it has been fun. In our competitive dog-eat-dog society the adrenaline rush has become too much a part of daily life. As in these two examples above, most people would not consider slowing down. It is bad enough that the stress of life regularly induces high levels of adrenaline in our bodies, which may be fun but is not healthy in the long run. What makes this problem more insidious is that we like this high a lot. The pleasure of the adrenaline response is habit forming.

When I went through medical school I encountered a famous textbook study that illustrated this phenomenon. Researchers implanted electrodes in the brains of rats and taught them to stimulate their own brains' pleasure center by either pressing one metal bar for food or another for a direct electrical stimulation to their pleasure center. The rats enjoyed the electrical self-stimulation so much that, when given the choice of food or electrostimulation of their pleasure centers, they went for the buzz. The rats eventually died from starvation. But they died happy.

The difference between the rats with electrodes implanted in their brains and you and me is that the output of adrenaline from the adrenal medulla is limited. When you persist in driving yourself, the constant demand you place on your adrenals will eventually cause your adrenals to fatigue. As your adrenals wear out, they will become increasingly less able to produce as much adrenaline in response to stimuli.

Imagine the following scenario. A citrus rancher named Simon Legree hires two pickers to harvest his orange crop. Throughout the first week the pickers continually harvest and bring Legree many bushels of oranges. The next week Legree is excited by his yield and decides that the pickers should keep on picking all night instead of having dinner and going to bed. So the next week the pickers pick all day and all night without rest or food. That week, they return with a smaller yield. Legree bellows at them that they must continue picking. By the end of the third week, the pickers' yield is yet smaller. Legree is panicked now because he needs those oranges, and he begins to berate and terrorize the pickers until they finally limp back to work. Exhausted and starving, they can only pick a few oranges a day. As the weeks go on, the pickers become so depleted and haggard that they cannot even reach up and pick one orange.

This is a metaphor for what happens to your adrenal glands when you get caught in the adrenaline rush lifestyle and do not allow your adrenal glands to rest and repair. When you reflected on Scout's story you may have thought about how much energy you used to have, how good you once looked and felt, and how soundly you used to sleep. It was because your adrenals were healthy and fully functioning back then. Although losing total adrenal function is rare, adrenal exhaustion—what you are probably suffering from to some degree now—is extremely common.* Adrenal fatigue affects all the interconnected systems of the body and creates a biological domino effect that causes fatigue, cravings, weight gain, mood swings, and many of the health problems people are grappling with today.

For those who love the lifestyle of the constant adrenaline rush, there is one more downside. When your adrenals tire and reduce their output of adrenaline, you will need more competition, more risk, more danger, more stimulus—more of the edge to get your adrenaline buzz. Paul Revere and the Raiders once sang: "Kicks just keep getting harder to find." Although you may place even greater demands on yourself to get the same response, eventually there is no more adrenal reserve. If you do not take measures to correct the situation, you may hit bottom emotionally and physically.

Ten years ago, at age forty-five, Rachel saw her business go into a decline and crash. "My husband and I lost everything that means anything in L.A. Before this happened we had a maid who came in every day and a live-in nanny for our daughter. I never saw the inside of my kitchen and I never did the laundry. I created a lifestyle in which I did

---

* An example of total adrenal failure is Addison's disease, a rare condition in which the adrenal glands fail to secrete stress hormones. Addison's is caused by the progressive destruction of the adrenal gland due to an infectious disease or from trauma such as a car accident, gunshot, or knife wound. It is possible to burn your adrenals out to this point, but it is not likely. People with Addison's disease must take adrenal hormone supplements prescribed by a physician. *The advice in this book is not intended as a substitute for the treatment by your doctor.*

not have to do the things that I thought were unnecessary for me to do and then suddenly I was *it*. I spent two years schlepping around the house in my sweats, depressed and doing laundry. Consulting jobs would come in every once in a while, so I could make some money. But I was devastated. I felt like a total failure and I didn't know how to get myself out of the basement."

It is not uncommon for the course of people's lives to correspond with fluctuations in their health. As Rachel persisted in squeezing the life out of her adrenals, and her adrenal reserve decreased, it is likely that her ability to keep her business afloat also diminished. It is typical of someone who loves the adrenaline rush to maintain a level of denial about what they are doing to themselves as their inner world begins to collapse. All of a sudden there is no fuel to maintain the same level of intensity or to handle adversity. As Rachel ran out of juice, so did the whole organization she was running.

It is also not uncommon to fall into a depression while withdrawing from years of intensely pleasurable adrenaline responses. When you place undue demands on your adrenals for an extended period of time, the feel-good neurotransmitter dopamine also declines. At the same time, your brain's dopamine receptors become desensitized to stimulation. Now no matter how much you stimulate these receptors, they are too dulled to fully respond. In her business, Rachel had needed increasing challenge, excitement, and risk to keep her on the edge. When her highly charged life came to a screeching halt, she padded around the house in her sweats with exhausted adrenals and depleted dopamine and sank into a bleak depression.

You may relate to patients who come in to see me and say, "I just don't know what to do. I have tried everything and nothing seems to work. I've been well all my life. How come I'm so exhausted? I'm getting sick all the time. I have no energy. I constantly crave sugar and caffeine. I don't understand it." What people do not realize is that they can progress through the stages of adrenal burnout and not realize what is happening inside their bodies until they start to feel ill.

When Rachel came to see me, I explained my program of Ten Simple Solutions, which would restore her adrenal function and possibly make her feel better than she had ever felt in her life.

Simple Solution 1: Eat, Eat, Eat, All Day Long
Simple Solution 2: Exercise Less
Simple Solution 3: Calm Your Central Nervous System
Simple Solution 4: Pay off Your Sleep Debt
Simple Solution 5: Let Go of Your Favorite Poison
Simple Solution 6: Supplement a Tired Food Chain
Simple Solution 7: Oxygenate Your Body
Simple Solution 8: Learn about Hidden Toxins
Simple Solution 9: Have Fun Every Day
Simple Solution 10: Cultivate SELF-fulfillment

Because these solutions are so simple, it was easy for Rachel to begin to make changes, one step at a time. Within a month she began to look and feel better. She was excited about starting over. "I was running on empty," Rachel admitted. "After I went to see Dr. Hanley I finally had the knowledge to help me get my body back together. I learned how to eat well and what vitamins and herbs to take. I began to build my resources back. Suddenly I got offered a job and I had to get dressed and get out of the house—and I was physically prepared to go out into the world again. I was looking pretty dried up and old before. Now I look in the mirror and I can see that I look younger. So I got back my health and my life." Like Rachel, here is what you can look forward to when you follow the simple solutions:

Lose weight

Increase your metabolism
Burn away fat around your
middle

Develop your ideal body composition
Lose cellulite

Gain power and control over your life

Quit habits such as nicotine, sugar, caffeine, and other stimulants

Feel calm and at peace

Have more patience

Stop being controlled by temper tantrums and emotional meltdowns

Feel more creative and productive

Have the emotional reserve to handle life's issues

Feel more pleasure

Gain renewed sense of satisfaction in life

Feel optimistic and positive about life and yourself

Have the energy to enjoy your family again

Remember what makes life worth living

Be more likely to accomplish your dreams and goals

Have the energy to enjoy the fruits of your success

Have more self-confidence

Enjoy better relationships

Be able to relax and stop sweating the small stuff

Sleep deeply and restfully every night

End insomnia

Instead of dragging around exhausted, have energy to burn

Stop nightmares and have pleasant dreams

Stop trekking to the bathroom all night long

Stop and even reverse accelerated aging

Improve concentration and mental clarity

Gain better short-term memory

Have thicker and shinier hair

Develop softer and smoother skin

Watch wrinkles disappear

Grow stronger nails

End dark circles under your eyes

Restore emotional stability

Feel safer and more secure

Get off your emotional roller
  coaster

End cravings

Feel happy and well
  adjusted

Stop obsessing, worrying,
  and feeling anxious

Feel the thrill of being healthy

Develop an increased sex
  drive

Increase fertility (for women)

Improve testosterone and
  sperm count (for men)

Have less aches and pains,
  fewer doctor visits

Rely less on prescription
  and over-the-counter
  drugs

Restore and improve immunity

Reduce occurrence of flu,
  cold and bronchitis

Have fewer allergies

Take fewer sick days

Diminish herpes outbreaks

Be on your way to freedom
  from arthritis

Prevent disease and early death

Reduce risk for cancer, heart
  disease, stroke, osteoporosis,
  neurological disorders—all
  of which are consequences
  of the adrenaline rush
  lifestyle

Reduce the tendency to
  develop osteoporosis

Live longer with better quality
  of life

Perhaps some of these benefits sound too good to be true, but I have seen the results thousands of times. All it takes are a few small changes.

The Five Stages of Adrenal Burnout

Denial will not make it go away

Most ambitious people have at one time or another stopped to think about what might happen if they kept driving themselves. For forty-seven-year-old Danielle Di Benedetto, it was the proverbial bad dream. She opened her eyes to a group of solemn-faced doctors gathered around her hospital bed. The chief of cardiac surgery cleared his throat and stoically delivered the prognosis. Her main coronary artery was 95 percent occluded; two other major arteries were 75 percent occluded. The doctors did not know if she would survive emergency triple bypass surgery. However, they were going ahead with the operation, and they gave her two days to notify her family and get her affairs in order. Danielle was stunned.

Danielle was an ambitious entrepreneur, yet she had been fully committed to living a healthy life for over ten years, including eating well, or so she thought, having regular massages and acupuncture and taking plenty of vacations. She could not imagine words like *arteriosclerosis, angina pectoris,* or *myocardial infarction* applying to her. What Danielle had not known is that, despite all of her healthy pursuits, she had been sowing the seeds of adrenal burnout for a very long time.

Behaviors that are the seeds of adrenal burnout

Skipping meals/dieting

Eating processed, junk, or fake foods

Not exercising or exercising too much

Avoiding or neglecting relaxation and other ways to calm your central nervous system

Not getting enough sleep

Blowing past your own fatigue to finish the day's work

Using sugar, caffeine, nicotine, drugs, or herbal stimulants to function at a higher rate when you are already tired

Breathing shallowly when tense, instead of breathing deeply

Exposing yourself to toxins through the environment, household products, and food

Worrying

Mentally replaying stressful inner dialogues

Neglecting fun and relaxing activities that allow you to clear your mind

Putting yourself last

You may be a perfectionistic mother who leaves little time for herself, an idealistic schoolteacher who works far too many hours, a student who is hyperfocused on getting and staying on the dean's list, or a computer techie who pulls all-nighters while trying to cash in on the Internet boom. Whatever your dream, it is possible, even probable, that like Danielle you are sowing the seeds of adrenal burnout without even realizing it.

Danielle is a tall, willowy redhead with intense green eyes and an expansive smile. Born and raised in New York, she launched her career blessed with inherent talent and drive. Danielle is a self-proclaimed hustler who has a golden touch. "Everything I tried in my career worked. At eighteen I had my own clothing boutique; at nineteen I had three boutiques. By twenty-four I was the junior designer for an elite fashion house. My successes went on like that, so I never could stop. Success was a blessing and a curse. I was hooked."

In addition to her driving career ambition, in her twenties after work Danielle flitted from one A-list party to the next or partied all night with the beautiful people. Smoking cigarettes and drinking coffee gave her an added lift to keep up the frantic pace. Wherever she went, she left a trail of candy wrappers.

Could this be you?

DRIVEN: You love taking risks and rising to challenges. You have great dreams and ambitions. You love an edgy, alert feeling. Everyday demands and self-imposed goals run you. You are always on the go. Occasionally you stay up very late at night or even pull all-nighters at work, school, with your newborn baby, or socializing. You have a lot of energy and are extremely productive. Because of these pressures and demands, you find you cannot exercise as much as you think you should—or you exercise to the extreme. You are turning to caffeine and sugar for energy. You may have taken up smoking cigarettes, perhaps thinking it gives you a boost. Even so, you feel and look great. Every day is an adventure that you look forward to. Life is a blur of activity, and you love it.

What you may not realize is that while you are engrossed in your happy and productive lifestyle, your body is scrambling to keep up. Every highly charged situation will cause an initial adrenaline rush. When the stress continues, the hormones cortisol and DHEA are next secreted from the adrenal cortex throughout the day and night to help your body function. The amounts of cortisol and DHEA that are secreted are altered and influenced by the degree of the intensity of your experiences. When your brain senses greater prolonged stress, such as staying up until 2 A.M. to meet a deadline, more cortisol and DHEA are secreted. When that need diminishes, as when you finally go home and go to bed, cortisol and DHEA levels decline. The

Figure 2
Cortisol and DHEA respond to all of life's chronic demands

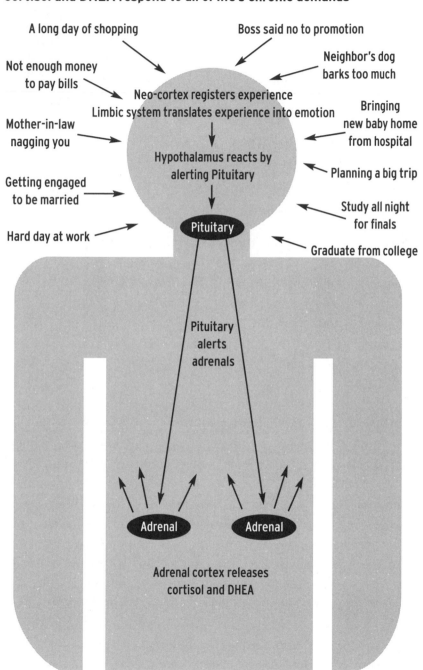

cortisol/DHEA response is good and healthy. During the Driven
stage, this response helps keep you going.

Healthy level of cortisol

Maintains blood sugar balance
Maintains energy
Maintains healthy blood pressure and fluid balance

Diminishes inflammation
Provides direction to the systems of the body
Regulates healthy immune
  response

Healthy level of DHEA

Decreases recovery time from
  exercise
Decreases the risk of cardio-
  vascular disease
Increases human growth
  hormone
Improves immunity

Improves mood
Increases energy
Increases fat burning
Is correlated with
  longevity
Speeds recovery from
  surgery

Cortisol and DHEA cannot bail you out indefinitely. Just as you
would not rev your car's engine 24/7, and just as you regularly maintain your car's engine, your body, and more specifically your adrenal
glands, need what I call Three Rs: Rest, Repair, and Rejuvenation.
When your body is given the opportunity to relax, biochemical
changes occur that foster the nourishment and rejuvenation of your
adrenals and your other vital organs. If your adrenal glands are constantly churning out stress hormones 24/7 and not given the opportunity to Rest, Repair, or Rejuvenate, their functional abilities will
diminish. You will begin to suffer from insomnia, fatigue, mood
swings, low sex drive, weight gain, water retention, and gastrointestinal discomforts, to name just a few problems.

As you continue to drive yourself, your adrenals will first decrease

DHEA production. Now you have too much cortisol and not enough DHEA. This is not a good situation because DHEA buffers many of the negative effects of excess cortisol. For example, cortisol causes muscle wasting, and DHEA stimulates muscle building, essentially replacing what cortisol has broken down. Increased cortisol suppresses immunity, whereas DHEA increases immunity. Increased cortisol leads to increased weight gain, whereas DHEA leads to fat burning and weight loss.

Taking DHEA supplements is not the only answer. Your body functions effectively when all of its systems operate in unison. Increasing DHEA to match an already high level of cortisol would only accelerate the damage to your adrenal glands.

Excess cortisol results in

Bone loss	Menstrual disorders
Decreased sex drive	Muscle wasting
Emotional mood swings— depression	Recurrent infections
	Slower wound healing
Increasing tendency to type II diabetes and hypertension	Thinning of the skin and connective tissue
	Water retention
Gastritis	Weight gain

Moving into her thirties, Danielle continued her hectic work life, smoking cigarettes, maintaining heavy sugar consumption, and not making time to rest or to eat balanced meals. Her first real physical difficulties began in this decade of her life.

At thirty-one, Danielle injured her spine. Perhaps her body was trying to tell her, "I *need* you to slow down and start paying attention because I can't keep up with you. If you don't start taking better care of me, things are going to go seriously wrong." Danielle did not hear or acknowledge these warnings. After recovering from her spinal injuries, even though she suffered from numbness in her legs, she did not stop working or even slow down her pace. "I was designing a ready-to-wear collection for an upcoming European fashion show. I spent a month working late nights standing up at my worktable, leaning over to work." Totally exhausted, she collapsed and reinjured her spine.

At this point, if Danielle had stopped to rest, her adrenal glands would have repaired themselves and been able to support her body. Instead, for the next five years Danielle depended on sugar, cigarettes, and cocaine, as well as prescription Quaaludes, muscle relaxants, codeine, and Valium, to get through her busy days.

Could this be you?

DRAGGING: You feel less energetic than you used to, so you jump-start your system in the morning with caffeine. During the day, you eat junk food, such as drive-through burgers and fries, and sugar, such as white flour products, including bread, bagels, pretzels, pasta, and donuts. You drink coffee or Diet Coke or use herbal stimulants such as ephedra or ma huang in an attempt to function at a higher rate. You may even occasionally turn to higher octane stimulants such as cocaine, Ritalin, Dexedrine, or other amphetamine-like drugs. At night, to relieve aches and pains or to relax, you may turn to ibuprofen, Pepto-Bismol, and/or Valium. If you took up smoking in your Driven stage, now you are probably "smoking more and enjoying it less." Occasional insomnia stalks you. You are getting a little flabby and growing love handles. Or maybe you are losing a little bit too much weight. But you can never be too rich or too thin, right? You keep a light attitude with yourself about losing your edge and getting older. You are not really worried. You have always come out all right and, after all, you are not getting older, you are getting better.

At this stage you really could improve your health, but unfortunately most people do not stop to rest, so their decline in health continues. One of the reasons for this steady decline is that when you do not allow your body time to Rest, Repair, and Rejuvenate, your body becomes too acidic as a result of remaining too long in what is known as the sympathetic state.

Your autonomic or unconscious nervous system, which regulates functions such as your intestines, heart, circulation, and glands, has two modalities: the sympathetic and the parasympathetic nervous systems. During the day, when you are awake, responding to stress, eating, and on the go, you are predominantly in the sympathetic state. This is when most of the critical metabolic processes take place within your body. It is appropriate and necessary to be in a sympathetic state part of the time because your body needs the operational metabolic processes that take place during this time. But people engage in behaviors that force their bodies into a constant state of sympathetic dominance. These behaviors, listed here, place constant extreme demands on your adrenal glands to secrete the stress hormones adrenaline, cortisol, and DHEA. This constant demand ultimately depletes your adrenal reserve.

Behaviors that result in a state of sympathetic dominance

Skipping meals/dieting

Eating processed, junk, or fake foods

Not exercising or exercising too much

Avoiding or neglecting relaxation and other ways to calm your central nervous system

Blowing past your own fatigue to finish the day's work

Not getting enough sleep

Using sugar, caffeine, nicotine, drugs, or herbal stimulants to function at a higher rate when you are already tired

Breathing shallowly when tense, instead of breathing deeply

Exposing yourself to toxins through the environment, household products, and food

Worrying

Mentally replaying stressful inner dialogues

Neglecting fun and relaxing activities that allow you to clear your mind

Putting yourself last

The metabolic processes that take place while you are in a sympathetic state create acids as byproducts, which make your body more acidic. Although these are natural and necessary processes, acid is not good for the body, and the body is not meant to stay in an acidic state. When your body is in a natural, healthy rhythm, the parasympathetic mode, which occurs predominantly at night, counteracts the sympathetic mode by turning on the repair processes. These processes rid your body of acid and tend to make your body more alkaline. An alkaline environment allows all the repair processes, such as making new cells, membranes, tissues, enzymes, hormones, and neurotransmitters, to continue.

It is too simple to say that your body moves from the sympathetic to the parasympathetic modes only in day and night, respectively. In every hour your body responds to millions of microinputs throughout your biochemistry. The ebb and flow of your acidic sympathetic and alkaline parasympathetic modes functions to maintain an extremely narrow range of pH within the body. Each input adjusts the ebb and flow of your sympathetic or your parasympathetic mode. It is like having your hands on the steering wheel of your car. You do not steer in an absolutely straight line—even if the road is relatively straight and smooth. You constantly make adjustments to the steering wheel. Likewise, your autonomic nervous system is constantly making adjustments from sympathetic to parasympathetic mode.

When your body's autonomic nervous system flows from the sympathetic mode to the parasympathetic mode, it is a time for your body to balance the day's acidity. This is known as the alkaline tide.

Before electricity, sitting by the light of a fire at night was a natural way for our ancestors' systems to change rhythm and to wind down from a day of work. When the fire burned out after a couple of hours humans went to sleep, and their bodies flowed gently into the alkaline tide, the natural repair and rejuvenation phase, when cells, membranes, tissues, hormones, enzymes, and neurotransmitters are regenerated. Unfortunately, modern humans engage in behaviors such as overwork, lack of rest, eating processed foods, and consuming caffeine and other stimulants that prevent a proper alkaline tide, and we become increasingly acidic.

The enzymes that direct metabolic processes—those processes that govern how your body functions—can only operate within a relatively neutral pH. When you live in an acidic state of sympathetic dominance, your body's enzymes cannot do their jobs properly, and numerous metabolic processes such as digestion, making energy, and repairing muscle are slowed down. Because the human body's processes are interdependent, one stalled process affects the next until your entire system becomes bogged down and sluggish. For example, when your digestive system is bogged down, nutrients do not get absorbed and your body has less regeneration and repair capabilities. You are likely to suffer from gastrointestinal problems such as esophageal reflux, bloating, gas, constipation, and irritable bowel. When your energy-making processes are stalled, your metabolism slows down. You are likely to gain weight, have less energy, and feel less creative and less excitement for life. When your body bogs down on rebuilding muscles, your heart could ultimately become less efficient in pumping blood through your system. This leads to fatigue, and you could ultimately suffer from congestive heart failure. These three examples demonstrate how premature aging occurs. When metabolic processes are stymied, intracellular trash called lipofucsin (*lipo few sin*) collects in your cells, damaging your system on a molecular level, accelerating the disease and the aging process.

At age thirty-six, Danielle quit smoking and gave up all stimulants. This was a great thing to do for her body. Unfortunately, Danielle did not slow down. "I was always on a fast train. While I was physically in one place I was mentally already at the next. No one could keep up with me. I didn't want to stop, and besides, I thought if life really wanted me to stop, it would stop giving me everything." True to form, Danielle packed even her mornings with activity, hiring a personal trainer to help her work out before dawn. She thought she was doing the right thing by exercising. But she was only getting four or five hours of sleep at night, which prevented her body from flowing into the alkaline tide to Rest, Repair, and Regenerate. Her body did not have enough time to wind down and fully enter a parasympathetic state of repair. Then, bouncing out of bed before she had a chance to repair launched her body back into a full sympathetic state. Danielle spent too many hours of the day and night in an acidic state of sympathetic dominance.

From age thirty-eight to forty-two Danielle served as the senior designer of another major fashion house. She had five assistants working under her. Four times a year she traveled from New York to Europe, where her lines were shown in Paris and Milan. Her appetite for fresh food was gone, and her cravings for sugar increased. She began to waste away until she was alarmingly thin. Her memory was foggy, and she could not contain her irritability.

On one such trip, as she returned from Paris, Danielle's plane was held up on the tarmac for two hours. During the flight Danielle suffered a severe allergic reaction to the jet fuel fumes she had been exposed to during the delay. Upon landing, Danielle was taken from the flight in a wheelchair. At that point, even *she* began to consider that there might be something terribly wrong.

Could this be you?

LOSING IT: You have dark circles under your eyes. Everything you eat seems to turn to fat, or you are wasting away to skin and bones. Either way, you are looking older. Insomnia is your regular bedfellow, and you often lie awake worrying about your day or what is coming the next day. Life is not what it used to be. Exercise is not a meaningful part of the equation. Instead, you grab whatever time you can on the couch. You are consuming coffee, sugar, and other stimulants throughout each day in an attempt to keep your edge. Possibly, the dozen times you tried to give up smoking haunt you, but you try not to think about it. It is hard for you to believe that you of all people are suffering from acute anxiety—with no immediate cause—shortness of breath, chest pains that could be mistaken for a heart attack, vertigo, palpitations, nausea, blurred vision, dread, the feeling that you will lose mental control, and/or feelings of impending death. It seems like all of a sudden you have environmental sensitivities, and you feel depressed and moody. In fact, you find yourself snapping at loved ones or colleagues, and this behavior shocks you. Although your blood tests are normal, you know there is something wrong. At the same time, you begin to wonder why you are working so hard. Antidepressants may appear to be your next step.

When Danielle realized that she was suffering from allergic reactions to chemicals in the environment, she quit her job and sought refuge on Martha's Vineyard, an island off the southwest coast of Cape Cod, Massachusetts. There, she went on a series of juice fasts for the next six months, which she believed healed her from her environmental sensitivities.

As soon as Danielle felt marginally better, she proceeded to create an industry out of juice fasting. She developed a fruit juice company and began consulting to a steady stream of entertainment celebrities and fashion moguls on the merits of juice fasting.

For the next four years, Danielle felt fluish, cranky, and bone tired. "People have always described me as someone who is full of life. But I didn't have the same passion for my life anymore. My irritability bothered me more than ever."

One morning she awoke and could not get out of bed. At forty-six Danielle had successfully reached the next stage of adrenal burnout.

Could this be you?

HITTING THE WALL: Your family and friends are fed up with hearing you gripe about how exhausted you are, how much you have to work, how much you hate your work—that you used to love—and how fat you are. A dense fog has settled over your memory, your emotional tantrums have escalated, and you cannot seem to take your mind off your worries. Insomnia, nightmares, gastrointestinal problems, allergies, asthma, headaches, migraines, musculoskeletal pains, back pain, and a stiff neck are all too familiar. Sleeping pills, antacids,

antiinflammatories, cholesterol-lowering medications, blood sugar–
lowering agents, and/or blood pressure medications have become a
way of life. The five to ten cups of coffee and/or caffeinated drinks
you drink are barely making it possible for you limp through the day.
At night, the only way to relax seems to be with a couple of drinks.
Your nocturnal treks to the bathroom are becoming increasingly frequent. It seems like fluids go right through you, and you wonder if
your bladder is shrinking. If you are taking antidepressants, they may
no longer be working. You are tense, worried, and frightened. Because you have not made time for hobbies and recreational activities,
you may be isolated from people, except for work and the occasional
obligatory cocktail party. You have no energy for socializing or even
for planning a vacation.

Think of your adrenal supply as a reservoir. Like any reservoir, when
its contents are being used, they must be replenished or the reservoir
will eventually run dry. Your adrenal reservoir is depleted by any of
the other behaviors that keep you in an acidic state of sympathetic
dominance. As you continue your habits, not realizing that you are
draining your precious adrenal reserves, your adrenal glands will
work overtime to keep up. In a constant state of sympathetic dominance your adrenal glands, weighing less than five grams each, will
actually grow as much as two grams in an attempt to meet the demand. This is a sign that your body can, to some degree, rise to meet
the need. When the demand continues and your adrenals have
reached maximum growth, their abilities and reserve will begin to
decline. Even so, they will keep working until they have atrophied
and their reservoir is practically dry. Just as you did not realize that
you were draining your adrenal reserves, you will likely not recognize
the symptoms until you are Hitting the Wall or Burned Out.

As you have been in the all-systems-go mode, the same behaviors
that have depleted your adrenal reserves have simultaneously depleted the reserves of the interconnected, interdependent systems of
your body. These systems include your entire endocrine system—
which is one of the major communication networks within your

body—your neurological system, and your immune system, to name a few. The human body has set standards that all its systems are designed to maintain in an attempt to keep the body's processes in a state of status quo, or homeostasis. Although these systems' reserves may be greatly depleted, they will continue to work erratically in an attempt to keep your body in balance.

Your body works best when it is humming along with all of its systems operating efficiently like a finely tuned engine. When your reserves are depleted and your systems are not operating at capacity, there are consequences: you seem to catch every virus that comes by, or you have an allergic reaction to something that never bothered

What happens to you when your adrenal reserves are depleted

Anxiety	Infertility
Arthritis	Insomnia, fatigue
Autoimmune diseases	Irrational fears
Chronic fatigue	Irregular menses
Colitis	Low sex drive
Depression	Metabolic problems
Eating disorders	Mood disorders
Escalating allergies, hives	Muscle spasms
Esophageal reflux	Palpitations
Fatigue	Premature heart disease
Fibromyalgia	Sciatica
Gastrointestinal dysfunction	Stiff neck
Headaches, migraines	Sweating (excessive)
Hypoglycemia and type II diabetes	Temporomandibular joint syndrome (TMJ)
Inability to make healthy cognitive choices	Water retention
Infections such as recurrent herpes, yeast, respiratory	Weight gain or weight loss

you. Now that your systems are working unreliably in fits and starts, chronic physical and emotional conditions, illnesses, and diseases are likely to get a foothold.

In 1997 at the end of Fashion Week in Paris, Danielle flew to Fiji for several weeks to relax. When she returned to New York, she began to notice a burning sensation in her chest. She had had problems in the past with bronchitis and pneumonia, and she attributed the discomfort to sensitive lungs and cold weather. She decided it was time to move west. Danielle settled in La Jolla, California. She was bone tired and committed to taking six months off work. Her morning walks in the hills became nearly impossible due to increased burning in her chest and shortness of breath.

Through a friend, Danielle, then forty-seven years old, ended up in my office in Malibu. She walked in and said, "I think I'm in menopause. I'm sweating all the time. I'm tired and cranky. I've always been too thin and now I'm gaining weight. I'm aging fast and I don't know what is going on." She did not tell me about her chest pain, but because of her family history of heart disease, I suggested she have an Ultra Fast CAT scan of her heart, which was a new test at the time.

Danielle was leaving the next day for New York and decided to postpone the test until she returned. "I got to New York and could not walk down three city blocks. I was leaning on buildings—my chest was burning. I went to a doctor who said, 'I'm not letting you out of the office until you take nitroglycerine, and you're not getting on the plane until you sign a release form, because you could have a heart attack any minute.' I said, 'Don't be ridiculous.'" Danielle left the doctor's office and booked a flight to the West Coast.

Back in California Danielle told me about her experience in New York with the "crazy" doctor. I insisted she go for the Ultra Fast CAT scan of her heart, a procedure that determines the level of artery calcification. Danielle's score was the highest the doctor had ever seen. "The doctor told me I was going to have a heart attack any minute. He said I could walk across the room and keel over and that 'It will be fatal.'" There was no more denying that Danielle had reached burnout—*at forty-seven years old.*

Could this be you?

BURNED OUT: This is crisis mode. You cannot get out of bed. You are snapping at the ones you love. Your creativity is long gone, and you have nothing left to give. You can barely remember what once made life worth living. Everything you do is a major effort. Although your doctor may say that your blood tests are normal, you know that there is something seriously wrong. You feel it. You are feverish, weak, achy. Or worse, cancer, heart attack, or chronic fatigue has reared its ugly head. Now that your immune system is depleted and behaving erratically, it can lose the ability to distinguish between normal healthy cells and destructive foreign invaders. An autoimmune disease is more likely to occur or be exacerbated, such as thyroiditis, lupus, Crohn's disease, rheumatoid arthritis, insulin dependent diabetes, Grave's disease, myasthenia gravis, interstitial cystitis, or Sjögren's disease, which causes dry eyes and mouth. You may have been involved in a major car or other potentially fatal accident that was the result of fatigue, depression, drinking, or drugs. You are not the same person you once were, and your family and friends cannot relate to you. You have never been so lonely.

For Danielle, who was used to being in control, having a catheter inserted into her bladder and being told she could not get out of bed even to pee was unbearable. In the two days before surgery, Danielle charmed her way into the hospital's Elizabeth Taylor suite. In addition to getting her affairs in order and notifying her friends and family, she choreographed elaborate plans for lunches and refreshments for the stream of supporters she penciled in for post-op visits. Underneath her drama queen façade, however, Danielle began to consider and reflect on what was truly important in her life and what was not.

The actual surgery was the ultimate reality check. The surgeons had told her that she would be back on her feet in six weeks, but six weeks after surgery it still hurt to breathe. Danielle was fragile and weak. Her arduous recovery lasted over a year. Her denial fading,

Danielle wanted desperately to sort out what had happened to her. "People asked me, 'How could you have had open-heart surgery after all the things you did to be healthy?' I didn't know," Danielle said. "I said it must have been stress. They were shocked, because I don't think people really believe that stress does these things even though they hear it all the time. They look at you and say, 'Yeah, yeah, if you're stressed, go to Cancun.'"

It is true that Danielle's stress was a primary contributing factor in her adrenal exhaustion, which ultimately led to heart disease. However, the path toward adrenal burnout is paved with more than stress. Danielle had lived on pure sugar for many years in the form of juice fasts. It has been known for decades that sugar, or foods that rapidly turn into sugar in the system, such as fruit juice, white flour, pasta, bagels, bread, cookies, and cake, increase the secretion of the hormone insulin. Prolonged high levels of insulin dramatically cause damage to the blood vessels, which results in heart disease. Although Danielle went on juice fasts in an attempt to be healthy, she was literally bathing her cells in sugar and insulin, which resulted in a continual demand on her adrenals to secret adrenaline, cortisol, and DHEA. This constant demand eventually depleted her adrenal reserve. She had also engaged in other behaviors such as overwork, lack of rest, eating candy, and consuming caffeine and other stimulants that contributed to depleting her adrenal reserve. As her adrenal reserve diminished, the interconnected systems of her body went into panic mode, trying to keep going. It was only a matter of time before the years of being in an acidic state of sympathetic dominance caught up with her.

Many of Danielle's old friends were shocked to hear about what had happened to her. "It was like I defected from their camp," Danielle reflected. "Most of my New York friends fell away. After my operation, their attitude was, come on already, get over it. When are you going back to work? I knew then why I left New York. If I had stayed, I would have dropped dead on a city street one day." Danielle's friends, who were adrenaline rush junkies themselves, did not want to face what had happened to Danielle and what could ultimately happen to them. Her loneliness during her recuperation is typical of the Burned Out stage.

The good news was that as Danielle followed my program of Ten Simple Solutions, she began to heal and her health improved. At age forty-nine, everything Danielle touches still turns to gold. Her second chance has given her the opportunity to enjoy activities, such as writing, gardening, and gourmet cooking, that she had previously ignored in the whirlwind of her life. "When your life passes before your eyes and you have two days to do your inventory, boy, you really see what matters and what doesn't. Three-quarters of the things that I thought were so important meant absolutely nothing when I thought I was going to lose my life."

Danielle's story illustrates how easy it is to slip from one stage to another and how denial prevents all of us from admitting what we are doing to ourselves. Even when the signs are blatantly apparent to others, we are usually blind to the clues and resist others' attempts to help us. Thirty-three-year-old Caitlin Takahashi is a rep for a film production company in Manhattan. She was working sixty to seventy hours per week and was developing symptoms of chronic fatigue. "From time to time my family and friends would mention that I was under a lot of stress and pushing myself too hard," Caitlin said. "One day my mother-in-law, in an attempt to be sympathetic, remarked, 'You know, you are under a lot of stress and stress can do this to you.' I turned around and practically bit her head off. 'If it were just stress don't you think I'd be able to do something about it? If it were that simple, I could just quit my job and then I'd feel fine.' Of course, I wasn't about to drop a successful career, or admit to being so frail that I couldn't stand a little stress. Pride and stubbornness sent me straight into denial." Sound familiar?

Over the years I have seen many people who love the adrenaline rush doing everything they can to squeeze the last drop of life out of their exhausted adrenals. Many people end up in situations similar to Danielle's before they finally realize what they are doing to themselves.

You may be far from a cataclysmic illness. You may be exhausted or chronically constipated or suffering from heartburn. Whatever your problems, you now have a better understanding of how the adrenaline rush lifestyle has kept you on the track toward adrenal burnout and what else can occur if you stay there too long. In addition to the sheer fun of rising to challenges and taking risks, we all have our own motivations for living an adrenaline rush lifestyle. Sometimes we are not even aware of what they are. Would you like to know what motivates you?

Psychogenes

What drives you

In childhood, just as we inherit our genetic characteristics from our parents, we learn our beliefs and fears about life and about ourselves. I call these beliefs and fears our psychogenes.

We either learn our psychogenes from our parents or they are instilled in us by early influences. The psychogene equation ultimately results in illness. Here is how that works: Let's say your parents believed that they were destined to be poor and feared poverty. This belief/fear was the setup for their psychogene equation.

Next comes the corresponding emotion. Your parent's psychogene led them to fret, worry, and obsess over their station in life.

Your parents then took action to appease that emotion. In an attempt to make themselves feel better, they worked two jobs and made sure you did your share of chores around the house. They instilled in you the value of hard work. They did not take vacations or eat in fancy restaurants. They never seemed to relax and enjoy their lives even as their bank account grew. Your mother suffered from migraine headaches, and your father had a bad back.

As a young adult you found yourself believing that you had to work hard or you would never have enough. Your belief led you to worry a little too much about job security and your future. You stayed on the dean's list in college and maintained a perfect 4.0 GPA. You went on to enjoy great success in life. You suffered from migraine headaches and a bad back.

You followed your parent's psychogene equation:

Belief/fear → leads to emotion → leads to action → leads to illness

Rachel Kantor, the fifty-two-year-old woman who moped around in sweats after her real estate business collapsed, remembered how she acquired her psychogenes. "My parents came from nothing and their goal was to give their children everything that *they* never had. I was never asked to achieve but, thanks to decades of therapy, soul-searching, and introspection, I now understand that their feelings of fear and desperation simply bled through from one generation to the other, as if passed from mother to child in the womb."

Rachel's parent's attitudes about success and achievement were the fuel that fired her ambitions. As an adult, Rachel settled in Los Angeles, "where the quest for money and fame is palpable and where life's focus is overtly targeted on strategies to amass your fortune and rise to power." Her early success in business only served to confirm her psychogenes.

Rachel believed that money and status equaled happiness and feared that she would be unhappy without them. That led to fear of failure → led to overwork and not eating → led to inability to keep going, financial ruin, and depression.

Forty-eight-year-old David Morrow is a businessman, writer, and lecturer. David is an athletic-looking man, considering his lifestyle. For the last twenty years he has steadily worked ten, fifteen, and even twenty-hour days. He can count the number of weekends he has taken off each year on one hand. Until recently, he has scheduled his time with little regard for his needs such as rest and relaxation. "There are a lot of historical factors extending throughout my youth that created a sense of insecurity when I wasn't working really hard at whatever I was doing. My brother and I learned that if the house wasn't spotless and presentable to other people, if our homework wasn't done, if our car wasn't washed, there were consequences. I ultimately developed a belief system that as long as I continued to work hard, possibly harder than anybody else, I would be safe from my father who could make my home life very unpleasant with tirades and harsh criticism."

David believed that working harder than anyone else guaranteed safety. His fear of negativity, tirades, and harsh criticism → led to apprehension that he was not doing enough → led to workaholic behavior → led to depression. David's rigid upbringing taught him that hard work created a sense of safety in the world. "Sure, it created a sense of safety," David said. "But it also drove me until I was completely fried. If I hadn't backed off, I think it would have killed me." Had David not recognized his psychogene and altered his behavior he could have ended up with a heart attack or stroke.

Twenty-five-year-old Jason Wilkes learned from his father that no matter how hard he is on himself, it is not hard enough. "It has never been an option for me to be anything less than a huge success," Jason said. "Growing up I knew that I was going to go to a good high school and a great college and then kick major butt in business and be successful like my uncles and my father, and make a name for myself and have a high place in society. Unfortunately I wasn't very ambitious in college. I got sidetracked by smoking too much pot and didn't really pursue school as hard as I should have. Graduating from college was a major reality check. I did a one-year job at an investment bank, answering phones, being an assistant. It was extremely humiliating. I felt that because my ambition kind of dipped in college I hit rock bottom."

It is true that using drugs dampens ambition and that Jason's performance in college suffered because of his drug use. At the same time Jason's interpretation of "not being very ambitious in college" was getting a 3.5 GPA at one of California's best universities. The humiliating experience of hitting rock bottom after college was earning $25,000 answering phones and being an assistant in an internationally known consulting firm. One year later Jason is earning close to six figures as a dot com sales rep, yet there remains his father's nagging voice in the back of his mind questioning whether he could be doing even *better* if he had only been more ambitious in college.

Jason believed that no matter how hard he tried, it would not be good enough. His fear of being thought of as inadequate → led to self-doubt about his accomplishments → led to working hard and regularly blowing off steam by drinking heavily with business associates → led to back muscle spasms.

Jason is still in the Driven stage. If he recognizes and alters his psychogenes now, he will probably have a healthy and vital future. If not, his equation could end up in depression and alcoholism.

Danielle, the entrepreneur who had triple bypass heart surgery at age forty-seven, believed that her self-worth was tied to success and achievement. Her fear that not gaining larger-than-life status would confirm that she was not valued → led to obsession over achievements → led to workaholic behavior → led to triple bypass surgery.

The Perfectionist

Let's take a close look at perfectionism—one of the most difficult psychogenes. In a quest for perfection, forty-seven-year-old Chrisy Morneault has kept up a frantic pace for twenty-five years. The Morneaults and their three daughters are always well groomed and neatly dressed. Their house in a Midwestern suburb is as picture perfect as a magazine layout. The backyard has an unreal quality, as if each blade of grass has been arranged to perfection. The garage is shipshape perfect. Every room in the house is immaculate and beautifully decorated. The inside of the refrigerator is germ free. Even the trash under the kitchen sink seems sanitized.

The Morneaults work hard at their home and at their other goals—even if it means staying up all night. "For many years we had a business cleaning offices," Chrisy said. "I worked my daytime job and then the whole family would clean offices from five to eleven at night. We would get a few hours of sleep and then start all over the next day. On weekends we would clean our own house and work on our own remodeling projects. We would stay up around the clock until they were done."

The Morneaults overstretched financially to make their house, family, and life look perfect. Clothing could not look worn, their cars could not look used, the yard could not look weathered. When the newness wore off an item, it was replaced. They continued buying and buying and fixing and fixing so that the exterior of their lives appeared perfect. Their goal is not necessarily materialism but perfection. To this end, the Morneaults do not take weekends off. "We have taken vacations, but then we work twice as hard before we go so that everything is perfect when we come home. When I leave my house on vacation I literally rake the carpets with a garden rake on my way out of the door so that when I come back home everything will be perfect. The kids aren't allowed to go back in even if they forgot something."

Two years ago the financial pressure to keep her perfect house of cards from collapsing drove Chrisy to extremes. "For one solid year I worked my daytime office job, then I would go home and try to sleep for three or four hours and then I would go to my next job on an assembly line from eleven at night to seven in the morning. I would shower and then go back to my daytime job." During that year, the Morneaults continued buying things for their home and working on the remodeling projects. On the outside, their life appeared perfect. "But we found that we couldn't keep the work pace up and everything started to slide. One day my neighbor stopped by and found me curled up on the kitchen floor in a fetal position. I was so tired, I just dropped there. I couldn't even talk." The pressure was too much for their marriage, which nearly broke apart. Bills had piled up that they could no longer juggle. The Morneaults were forced to file for bankruptcy protection, and the house of cards of perfectionism came toppling down.

Chrisy understands how she became a perfectionist. "Since I was very little, I grew up cleaning and straightening things up—it was a family thing," Chrisy said. "It was mostly because of my mother. I always wanted to keep things looking good so that it wouldn't cause her to flip out. It was like we didn't want to give her any reasons." Chrisy's mother's drinking and suicide attempts, which began when Chrisy was seven, were the source of great anxiety in the family. Not that keeping the house perfect always kept Chrisy's mother calm. She would sometimes "flip out" even if the house was clean and ordered.

Chrisy believed that there was safety in perfection, and her fear of imperfection → led to anxiety, nervousness, and jitters when things were not perfect → led to blindly driving herself → led to nervous breakdown and bankruptcy.

Perfectionists are the ultimate never-enough personalities. If perfectionism is wreaking havoc on your health and standing in the way of happiness, the first hurdle is to recognize the fact that you are a perfectionist.

How to recognize if you are a perfectionist

____You will put any amount of energy into the details of a project, wanting everything to be just so

____You have many ambitious goals that you try to accomplish simultaneously

____You almost never finish everything you expect to accomplish in one day

____You do not feel a sense of satisfaction when you accomplish a goal, but rather you pick it apart for its flaws or you are already thinking of something else that needs to be done

____You never feel satisfied with yourself

____You are self-critical and unforgiving of your flaws

____You are compelled to work rather than do something fun

____Even when you are doing something that is supposed to be fun you turn it into a project/work

____You feel nervous taking time away from work, even if it is for family fun

____No matter what you do you feel that it is never enough

____You do not feel that you have high expectations of yourself or that you make unreasonable demands on yourself even though others tell you that you are too hard on yourself

If you checked three or more, you are probably a perfectionist. The next step is to admit how exhausting, depleting, and defeating your quest for perfection is and that no matter how perfect you become, you will never satisfy your own critical voice. Perfectionists often set self-defeating goals. "I always think that I am going to have more hours during the day to get things done," Chrisy said. "I might have ten jobs on a mental list that I think should be done that day. Maybe I get five of them done and then I get really depressed that I didn't get the other five done because I think that I should have been able to fit all of those into my twenty-four-hour day."

When it comes to change, we all need easy objectives. When we set reachable goals we can see and feel good about incremental progress, which makes us feel better about our lives and ourselves. Making successful changes gives us the incentive to attempt even more changes. No matter what psychogene drives you, change is a step-by-step process. Even small steps will take you closer to your goal. This is why I designed the Ten *Simple* Solutions.

These Simple Solutions will do more than change the exterior of your life. You can influence your biochemistry as well. In fact, you have more control over what goes on inside your body than you may believe.

You Can Influence Your Body's Biochemistry

When I went to medical school it was believed that a human being consisted of two separate entities, mind and body. The mind was thought to consciously control functions such as the musculoskeleton system, allowing us to flex our muscles and move our arms at will. Other processes of the body, such as our heartbeat, the secretion of hormones, the regulation of antibodies by our immune system, and so on were viewed as completely out of our conscious sphere of influence. It was believed that one could not cross the chasm between the mind and body. This belief has changed radically, thanks to the field of psychoneuroimmunology (PNI) (*sigh ko nur-o im you nol agee*), which studies the relationships that exist between the central nervous system, the autonomic nervous system, the endocrine system, the immune system, and the mind. The study of PNI has helped us understand that our thoughts and beliefs can influence our heart rate, blood pressure, digestion, and immunity and ultimately all of our bodily functions. This is exactly what a lie detector is based on. PNI has demonstrated that the mind and body are not only linked but are one and the same.

Your body's biochemistry is heavily influenced by what you think, feel, and believe. It is not so black and white that we can say that X belief or fear produces Y neurotransmitter, which leads to Z illness. There is no set equation that we can say results in a specific neurotransmitter being created. We do know that if we think enough negative thoughts, we will create unhealthy neurotransmitters that will result in mental depression and illness. For example, if you continually think *I am not safe in the world unless I work constantly,* this belief will deplete healthy, calming neurotransmitters. With fewer calming neurotransmitters, your beliefs and fears can run wild.

On the other hand, if you think *I am safe in the world, even when my work is not completely finished* or *I am happy because I set realistic goals and accomplished them,* you are likely to produce mood-elevating, healthy neurotransmitters, which will produce a feeling of well-being and safety. When acting out of a sense of safety, your self-confidence will allow you to behave in healthy ways, which will further enhance your health and vitality.

Your psychogenes have developed and been reinforced over the years. You have grown comfortable with and reliant on your habits and beliefs. If you have spent twenty years believing something to be true, you are not going let go of that belief/fear overnight. But changing your psychogenes is possible. For example, you may believe that you are incompetent and fear making mistakes, and this belief/ fear may make you feel panicky. It may be true that you believe these things about yourself and that your feelings are real. Changing your beliefs can only occur through changing your behaviors. Recognize first that your behaviors have never really made you feel better. In other words, if you feel inadequate, did workaholic behavior ever make you feel less so? Probably not. Working too hard only leads to ill health and less competency in the long run.

It is time now to engage in healthy behaviors, one step at a time, that will lead to a true sense of self-worth and self-esteem. As you change your behaviors, you will change your neurotransmitters too. Your new healthy neurotransmitters operating within your body will make it easier for you to make even more healthy changes. Here are a few variations on the unhealthy psychogene equation from some of my patients:

Your belief that you are inadequate and your fear of failure → leads to lack of self-confidence → leads to overwork/lack of sleep → leads to severe physical and emotional consequences

Your belief that you must never let your guard down or "let them see you sweat" and your fear of being found out → leads to worrying and fretting over your performance → leads to driving yourself relentlessly → leads to severe physical and emotional consequences

Your belief that being thin makes you better and your fear of being fat → leads to self-loathing → leads to yo-yo dieting → leads to severe physical and emotional consequences

Your belief that your worth hinges on success, power, money, and status and your fear of not achieving this status → leads to anxiety about your level of achievement → leads to workaholic behavior → leads to severe physical and emotional consequences

Your belief that you are stupid and your fear of life's challenges → leads to worrying yourself sick over your perceived mistakes → leads to making bad decisions → leads to severe physical and emotional consequences

Your belief that you should not show your emotions and your fear that showing your feelings will make you look incompetent → leads to panic and self-doubt → leads to saying yes to everything people ask of you → leads to severe physical and emotional consequences

Your belief that you are the provider and your fear of showing frailty → leads to anxiety that your family will not get what they need →

leads to working overtime even when your family needs you → leads
to severe physical and emotional consequences

What is your psychogene equation?

_____→ led to

What is your psychogene—your beliefs and fears?

_____→ led to

What emotion can you identify with your psychogene?

_____→ led to

What behaviors have you developed in an attempt to appease
that emotion?

_____

What emotional or physical symptoms have you developed
as a result?

Dramatic changes in a person's longstanding behavior do not
come easily or quickly. In fact, change usually occurs in small doses,
one step at a time. The process of changing behavior begins with
wanting to change. And we usually change when we get tired of suffering. You know it is time for a change when:

____ You are ready to go back to the way you used to be when you
     enjoyed life and felt optimistic
____ You want to feel good and vital again like you used to
____ You regret the closeness you have missed out on with your
     family
____ You are fed up with your own irritability
____ You want to stop your emotional meltdowns, such as losing
     control of your temper and behaving irrationally, shouting
     in the telephone, cutting people off in traffic, behaving
     rudely and/or insensitively and/or having crying jags

___ You want to find a better way of eating because you can no longer skip meals without feeling sick, lightheaded, and more apt to make errors in judgment

___ You have been yo-yo dieting and you are heavier than ever

___ You have been on a low-fat, high-carbohydrate diet and you are heavier and sicker than you were before

___ You realize that you are drinking too much coffee, eating too much sugar, and/or taking too many other stimulants— and you want to stop

___ You are ready to quit smoking

___ Your insomnia is really getting to you, and the fatigue, body aches, and mood swings have become unbearable

Now that you know what drives you, and you want to change, the next step is to determine where you are in the stages of adrenal burnout. Below is an easy-to-take adrenal reserve test on work, life, and dietary behaviors. Your score will help place you in one of the Five Stages of adrenal burnout so that you can follow the simple solutions tailored to your stage, found at the end of every chapter. If you are interested in clinical adrenal testing, please refer to the appendix for information on blood, urine, and saliva testing.

In the following test, to determine where you are in the Five Stages of Adrenal Burnout, check one response that *most* applies to you. Be as honest with yourself as possible—even if the truth hurts. As you evaluate these questions, factor in your behaviors over the last twelve months.

Your diet

How often do you crave sugar such as candy, sodas, popcorn, bagels, pasta, chips, cookies, pastries?
Does not apply ___   A few times a year or less ___   Up to twice a month ___
Up to twice a week ___   Every day or almost every day ___

How often do you crave salt?
Does not apply ___   A few times a year or less ___   Up to twice a month ___
Up to twice a week ___   Every day or almost every day ___

How often do you skip meals?
Does not apply ___   A few times a year or less ___   Up to twice a month ___
Up to twice a week ___   Every day or almost every day ___

Do you gain weight for no apparent reason?
No ___   Yes ___

Do you diet and lose weight only to regain it?
No ___   Yes ___

Do you diet but are unable to lose weight?
No ___   Yes ___

Use of stimulants

How often do you crave chocolate or candy?
Does not apply ___   A few times a year or less ___   Up to twice a month ___
Up to twice a week ___   Every day or almost every day ___

How often do you drink coffee and/or caffeinated drinks?
Does not apply ___   A few times a year or less ___   Up to twice a month ___
Up to twice a week ___   Every day or almost every day ___

How often do you drink alcohol?
Does not apply ___   A few times a year or less ___   Up to twice a month ___
Up to twice a week ___   Every day or almost every day ___

How often do you smoke cigarettes?
Does not apply ___   A few times a year or less ___   Up to twice a month ___
Up to twice a week ___   Every day or almost every day ___

How often do you use natural stimulants such as ephedra or ma huang?
Does not apply ___   A few times a year or less ___   Up to twice a month ___
Up to twice a week ___   Every day or almost every day ___

How often do you use legal or illegal stimulants such as Ritalin, cocaine, Dexedrine, ephedrine (or over-the-counter diet drugs), or other amphetamine-like drugs?
Does not apply ___   A few times a year or less ___   Up to twice a month ___
Up to twice a week ___   Every day or almost every day ___

Use of prescription or over-the-counter drugs

How often do you take over-the-counter medications such as ibuprofen, Tums, Sudafed, or Pepto-Bismol?
Does not apply ___   A few times a year or less ___   Up to twice a month ___
Up to twice a week ___   Every day or almost every day ___

How often do you take sleeping pills?
Does not apply ___   A few times a year or less ___   Up to twice a month ___
Up to twice a week ___   Every day or almost every day ___

How often do you take Valium or other tranquilizers?
Does not apply ___   A few times a year or less ___   Up to twice a month ___
Up to twice a week ___   Every day or almost every day ___

Do you take cholesterol-lowering medications, hypoglycemic agents, and/or blood pressure medications?
No ___   Yes ___

Do you take antidepressants?
No ___   Yes ___

Your life

How often does rising to challenges and taking risks give you a sensation of pleasure?
Does not apply ___   A few times a year or less ___   Up to twice a month ___
Up to twice a week ___   Every day or almost every day ___

Do you love the feeling of butterflies in your stomach and the thrill of taking chances?
Does not apply ___   A few times a year or less ___   Up to twice a month ___
Up to twice a week ___   Every day or almost every day ___

How often do you feel that you cannot do what you want because you must be responsive to the needs of others?
Does not apply ___   A few times a year or less ___   Up to twice a month ___
Up to twice a week ___   Every day or almost every day ___

How often do you push past stress or fatigue to accomplish your goals?
Does not apply ___   A few times a year or less ___   Up to twice a month ___
Up to twice a week ___   Every day or almost every day ___

How often do you allow your calendar and the lists you make to dictate how you spend your time?
Does not apply ___   A few times a year or less ___   Up to twice a month ___
Up to twice a week ___   Every day or almost every day ___

Have you gotten away from socializing with friends in lieu of working and meeting other obligations?
No ___   Yes ___

Is your personal life low on your list of priorities?
No ___   Yes ___

Do you party into the morning hours or even all night?
No ___   Yes ___

Your Work

As you reach a goal, how often do you find that you cannot enjoy your success because another, even larger goal is demanding your immediate attention?
Does not apply ___   A few times a year or less ___   Up to twice a month ___
Up to twice a week ___   Every day or almost every day ___

How often do you feel attached to your phone, pager, cell phone, or email?
Does not apply ___   A few times a year or less ___   Up to twice a month ___
Up to twice a week ___   Every day or almost every day ___

How often do you work late hours and/or on weekends?
Does not apply ___   A few times a year or less ___   Up to twice a month ___
Up to twice a week ___   Every day or almost every day ___

How often do you work all night?
Does not apply ___   A few times a year or less ___   Up to twice a month ___
Up to twice a week ___   Every day or almost every day ___

How often do you feel impatient or irritated when your children, spouse, or others interfere with your work time?
Does not apply ___   A few times a year or less ___   Up to twice a month ___
Up to twice a week ___   Every day or almost every day ___

Do you get sick when you take a vacation?
No ___   Yes ___

Do you take two weeks of vacation every year?
No ___   Yes ___

Are you unable to take vacations because you feel guilty about taking time off and/or just will not let yourself stop working?
No ___   Yes ___

Physical and emotional symptoms

How often do you experience any of the following symptoms: acute anxiety—with no immediate cause; shortness of breath; chest pains that could be mistaken for a heart attack; vertigo; palpitations; nausea; blurred vision; dread; the feeling that you will lose mental control; and/or feelings of impending death?
Does not apply ___   A few times a year or less ___   Up to twice a month ___
Up to twice a week ___   Every day or almost every day ___

How often do you feel like you are never enough, never doing enough, never good enough?
Does not apply ___   A few times a year or less ___   Up to twice a month ___
Up to twice a week ___   Every day or almost every day ___

How often do you peter out around 3 P.M. and reach for a stimulant—even just sugar—for energy?
Does not apply ___   A few times a year or less ___   Up to twice a month ___
Up to twice a week ___   Every day or almost every day ___

How often, when you bend down and when standing up, do you feel lightheaded or see stars?
Does not apply ___   A few times a year or less ___   Up to twice a month ___
Up to twice a week ___   Every day or almost every day ___

How often do you feel dizzy, faint, or momentarily weak?
Does not apply ___   A few times a year or less ___   Up to twice a month ___
Up to twice a week ___   Every day or almost every day ___

How often do you awaken in the morning exhausted?
Does not apply ___   A few times a year or less ___   Up to twice a month ___
Up to twice a week ___   Every day or almost every day ___

How often do you experience sudden shifts in temper?
Does not apply ___   A few times a year or less ___   Up to twice a month ___
Up to twice a week ___   Every day or almost every day ___

If you are a woman, how often do you suffer from PMS, perimenopause, or menopausal symptoms such as cravings, fatigue, edema, irritability?
Does not apply ___   A few times a year or less ___   Up to twice a month ___
Up to twice a week ___   Every day or almost every day ___

How often do you get colds and flu?
Does not apply ___   A few times a year or less ___   Up to twice a month ___
Up to twice a week ___   Every day or almost every day ___

How often do you get infections such as herpes, shingles, sinusitis, colitis, yeast, or boils?
Does not apply ___   A few times a year or less ___   Up to twice a month ___
Up to twice a week ___   Every day or almost every day ___

How often do you get constipated?
Does not apply ___   A few times a year or less ___   Up to twice a month ___
Up to twice a week ___   Every day or almost every day ___

How often do you get diarrhea?
Does not apply ___   A few times a year or less ___   Up to twice a month ___
Up to twice a week ___   Every day or almost every day ___

How often do you feel exhausted after exercise instead of exhilarated?
Does not apply ___   A few times a year or less ___   Up to twice a month ___
Up to twice a week ___   Every day or almost every day ___

How often do you suffer from insomnia?
Does not apply ___   A few times a year or less ___   Up to twice a month ___
Up to twice a week ___   Every day or almost every day ___

How often you feel uncomfortably cold, especially your hands and feet?
Does not apply ___   A few times a year or less ___   Up to twice a month ___
Up to twice a week ___   Every day or almost every day ___

How often you suffer from poor digestion, allergies, asthma, headaches, migraines, or musculoskeletal pains?
Does not apply ___   A few times a year or less ___   Up to twice a month ___
Up to twice a week ___   Every day or almost every day ___

How often do you have a short fuse with coworkers, family, and people in the service industries—such as waiters, hotel clerks, store clerks, and airline representatives—and shout in the telephone, cut people off in traffic, behave rudely and/or insensitively, and/or have a crying jag?
Does not apply ___   A few times a year or less ___   Up to twice a month ___
Up to twice a week ___   Every day or almost every day ___

How often do you suffer from short-term memory loss or confusion?
Does not apply ___   A few times a year or less ___   Up to twice a month ___
Up to twice a week ___   Every day or almost every day ___

How often does exercise take more from you than it gives you?
Does not apply ___   A few times a year or less ___   Up to twice a month ___
Up to twice a week ___   Every day or almost every day ___

How often do you resolve to exercise and then give up without much effort?
Does not apply ___   A few times a year or less ___   Up to twice a month ___
Up to twice a week ___   Every day or almost every day ___

How often, when you have free time, are you too tired to do anything else but vegetate?
Does not apply ___   A few times a year or less ___   Up to twice a month ___
Up to twice a week ___   Every day or almost every day ___

How often do you snap at innocent people—even when you feel your temper is justified?
Does not apply ___   A few times a year or less ___   Up to twice a month ___
Up to twice a week ___   Every day or almost every day ___

How often do you feel anxious?
Does not apply ___   A few times a year or less ___   Up to twice a month ___
Up to twice a week ___   Every day or almost every day ___

How often do you feel depressed, helpless, and/or hopeless?
Does not apply ___   A few times a year or less ___   Up to twice a month ___
Up to twice a week ___   Every day or almost every day ___

Do you trek to the bathroom two, three, four, five, or more times a night?
No ___   Yes ___

Do you have dark circles under your eyes? Ask a friend to tell you and to be honest.
No ___   Yes ___

To determine your score:

0 points for each "Does not apply" or "No" (for yes/no questions)

1 point for each "A few times a year or less" ___

3 points for each "Up to twice a month" ___

5 points for each "Up to twice a week" ___

7 points for each "Every day or almost every day" ___

7 points for each "Yes" (for yes/no questions) ___

Total ___

If you have any doubts about the accuracy of your score, put this test aside for a few days and come back to it with a fresh perspective.

If your score is 0 to 60: Congratulations. Everyone can improve, but obviously you are doing most things right. So keep doing what you are doing.

61 to 100 are scores typical of the Driven stage.

DRIVEN: You love taking risks and rising to challenges and big dreams and ambitions. You love the adrenaline rush. You may have started a few bad habits like eating junk food and sugar. But you still feel and look great. Life is a blur of excitement and energy.

There are financial, psychological, and social rewards for being driven, responsible, productive, and successful. If you recognize yourself in this category, and if you make some changes now by following the Ten Simple Solutions, you can maintain your energy level and your passion for life indefinitely.

101 to 150 are scores typical for the Dragging stage.

DRAGGING: You feel less energetic than you used to. Caffeine, junk food, and sugar are part of your daily diet. You may turn to an occasional over-the-counter drug or two when you have an ache or pain. Your sleep is not as sound as it was, and you are getting a little flabby—or you might be losing a little bit too much weight. But you are not worried yet.

The rewards, admiration, and respect you have achieved are the golden hand-cuffs that keep you going. At this point, you may be able to get off the track toward burnout with willpower and the help of the Ten Simple Solutions. You may not be aware of it, but you are inches away from more serious problems. Although there is still time for you to reassess your life and reprioritize, it is even more important at this stage that you recognize and temper the behaviors that will lead to adrenal burnout. Begin now to develop healthy, self-nurturing habits.

151 to 200 are scores generally indicating that you are Losing It.

LOSING IT: You have to admit you have dark circles under your eyes now. You really are too fat or too thin. Either way you are looking older. Insomnia is your chronic bedfellow, and you often lie awake worrying about what you have to do, what has been done to you, and what you still need to accomplish. Life is not what it used to be. Exercise is not much of a part of your life. Instead you rely too much on coffee, sugar, and other stimulants. You have been a grouch lately, and this behavior shocks you. You feel achy all the time as if you are on the verge of the flu, and you know there is something wrong. But nothing shows up on your medical tests.

You are too exhausted to bask in the pleasure of the rewards, admiration, and respect you have earned. You keep jamming and stuffing and cramming activity into your life so that you are like a drawer with a jumble of things hanging out of it. It is time to clean your inner and outer desktop, to delete what needs to be thrown away, and to reevaluate and reorder your priorities. It is time to make time for yourSELF. It will only become more difficult if you wait. You still have the strength to change the behaviors that will lead to adrenal burnout and to begin to develop healthy, nurturing habits. Please take your pedal off the metal now and operate at a pace that is consistent with regaining your health. Start to explore, incorporate, and experience the Ten Simple Solutions and discover how well you can feel.

201 to 250 are scores indicating you are Hitting the Wall.

HITTING THE WALL: Your family and friends are fed up with hearing you gripe about how exhausted you are, how much work you have to do, how much you hate your work, and how fat you are. Your memory is shot, you are having a lot of emotional tantrums these days, and you have an obsessive tape running in your brain. Insomnia, nightmares, gastrointestinal problems, allergies, asthma, headaches, migraines, musculoskeletal pains, back pain, and a stiff neck are all too familiar— along with the prescription and over-the-counter drugs you take to try to find relief. Caffeine and alcohol are pretty constant now. You have no energy and no real social life. Even so, you still doubt whether your behaviors are really affecting your health *that* much.

Do not pass go, because there is no longer $200 to collect. The rewards, admiration, and respect you have achieved are golden handcuffs that keep you going—even though you can barely stand it anymore. You may not be aware, but you are inches away from more serious problems. Now is your last chance to reassess your life and reprioritize before you reach Burned Out. Start to explore and discover how well you can feel. It is possible to develop healthy, self-nurturing habits—and you can do it.

251 plus are scores of the Burned Out.

BURNED OUT: This is crisis mode. You can barely remember what once made life worth living. You are feverish, weak, achy. Or worse, cancer, heart attack, or chronic fatigue has reared its ugly head. You may be suffering from an autoimmune disease. You may have been involved in a major car or other potentially fatal accident that was the result of fatigue, depression, drinking, or drugs, or you may have become an alcoholic or a drug addict. You have never been so lonely.

You probably cannot even recall the pleasure you once got from the rewards, admiration, and respect that you received for being driven. Society more or less ignores you now that you have hit bottom. If you do not die during this stage, there is no place to go but up.

Now that you know where you stand, part II outlines Ten Simple Solutions that will gently help you move backward in these stages. As you read these chapters, keep in mind that every simple solution is a suggestion offered to you as an option for you to explore. Some of these will be manageable for you right away; others you will grow into. The Ten Simple Solutions are designed to assist you in healing and nourishing your adrenal glands and to keep you from progressing any further down the path toward burnout. As you successfully incorporate the Simple Solutions into your life, you will experience your psychogenes and neurotransmitters changing. You will begin to enjoy the cascading effect of good health and happiness.

Part Two

Ten Simple Solutions

Simple Solution 1
Eat, Eat, Eat,
All Day Long

Graze your way to weight loss

Shortcuts to Simple Solution 1

- To lose weight, stop dieting.

- Eat regular balanced meals of real, whole foods.

- Do not eat processed, junk, and fake foods.

It is three o'clock in the afternoon. Forty-seven-year-old Chrisy Morneault has been going strong since five A.M., but she has yet to eat anything. "I'm not a breakfast person," she says. "When I wake up I just have coffee. I get home from my part-time job around one o'clock in the afternoon. I have to start supper then because the rest of the family starts getting home around three-thirty and they all want to eat. If I eat something, it is usually junk, like potato chips or a HoHo. It's the first thing that I can pick up and put into my mouth."

The Blood Sugar Roller Coaster

Whether or not you take time to eat, your body strives to maintain balanced blood sugar levels at all times. If your blood sugar were to fall too low for too long, you would slip into a coma. If your blood sugar remained too high for too long, you would develop type II diabetes. When you feel hunger pangs, your brain is telling you that your blood sugar is low and that you need to eat something right now. We all know the weak and light-headed feeling we get from not eating. If we persist in not eating, we can suffer gnawing hunger pangs and feel panic, anxiety, fatigue, exhaustion, cravings, and mood swings. Yet skipping meals is common—and people learn to live with these feelings.

Like many people, Chrisy's priorities do not include feeding herself. "If I knew that there were some things that I could do that were simple, I would like to try to make some changes," she commented. "By easy I mean that it wasn't complicated—like having to fix an egg for breakfast or make a salad every day for lunch." In other words, Chrisy will stay up all night wallpapering a bathroom, but cooking an egg is too complicated. Likewise, many people will get up before dawn to check the stock market, work until all hours of the night on a project for work or church, or get their kids fed and organized before they leave for school. But they will not remember, or think it is important enough, to feed their own bodies.

While you may not be interested in taking the time to eat, your brain is very concerned with having its tightly regulated supply of sugar (fuel). When you do not eat, it assumes that you are in a time of famine and sends a red alert to your adrenals to release adrenaline and cortisol. Adrenaline releases emergency energy from sugar stored in your liver and muscles, and cortisol *breaks down your own muscle mass* to turn it into sugar. Since excess sugar damages brain and body cells, this influx of sugar into your bloodstream triggers the secretion of insulin, which immediately stores this sugar safely away into cells as fat.

As long as you do not eat, your brain will continue to send red alerts to your adrenals. This adrenaline/cortisol/insulin vicious cycle of breaking down and storing away sugar will repeat over and over. This is a blood sugar roller coaster.

Figure 3
Blood sugar roller coaster

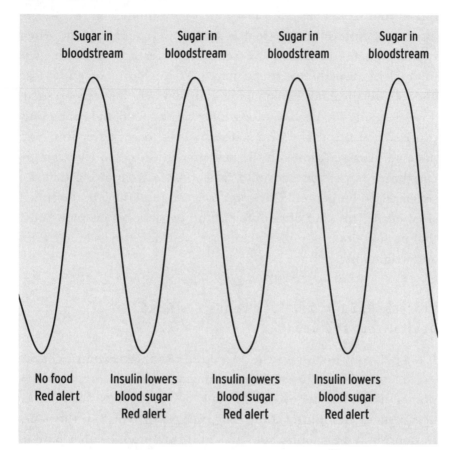

Restricting Food Will Make You Gain Weight

In addition to skipping meals, many people severely limit food portions in an attempt to lose weight. "I feel that in order to lose weight I have to starve myself," Chrisy says. "I usually eat soup and try to keep my intake to eight hundred calories a day." Chrisy's method of dieting by eating a bowl of canned soup at the end of a very busy day is a painful illustration of how many people view portion control. Although Chrisy has occasionally lost weight by starving herself this way, she is the first to admit that the weight does not stay off and she has been up to sixty pounds overweight for over twenty years.

When you severely limit your food intake, cortisol continually breaks down your own muscle mass. Since muscle mass dictates the rate of your metabolism, if you regularly go without food you are going to have diminished muscle mass and a lowered metabolism. When you finally get around to eating, with your lowered metabolism, your food will be turned into fat and stored. That is why people who lose and gain weight always end up fatter than they were when they started.

Restricting food is bad enough. Restricting food and eating only processed, junk, or fake food is disastrous. A recent cover story in a national news magazine, on the epidemic of obesity in children, focused on the portion sizes of a fast-food meal—implying that the smaller-sized burger and Coke and fries was preferable to the super-sized meal. This kind of misinformation perpetuates people's belief that portion control, rather than *what* you eat, is the issue to health and weight loss.

Processed, Junk, and Fake Foods Are Dead, Devitalized, and Deadly

It is a sad irony that we live in one of the wealthiest countries of the world, yet millions of us of all economic means suffer from malnutrition because of eating processed, junk, and fake foods. These products are devoid of nutrients and dietary enzymes to provide the basics to nourish and alkalinize your system. Many products that pose as food are so laden with chemicals and devoid of nutrition that bugs cannot even live on them. The chemicals, food additives, and preservatives in processed, junk, and fake foods have been linked to behavioral disorders, violence, hyperactivity, learning disorders, headaches, irritability, fatigue, ADD, ADHD, and cancer. These foods also contain an abundant amount of sugar and sodium which inhibit satiety and perpetuate cravings, leading to obesity and type II diabetes.

Processed, junk, and fake foods also contain toxic chemicals, pesticides, and damaged fats. These food products *are not real food*—they are dead, devitalized, and deadly. In fact, it is a dangerous experiment that humans are living on processed, junk, and invented foods that have never before existed as part of our food chain.

Figure 4
Dieting makes you fatter

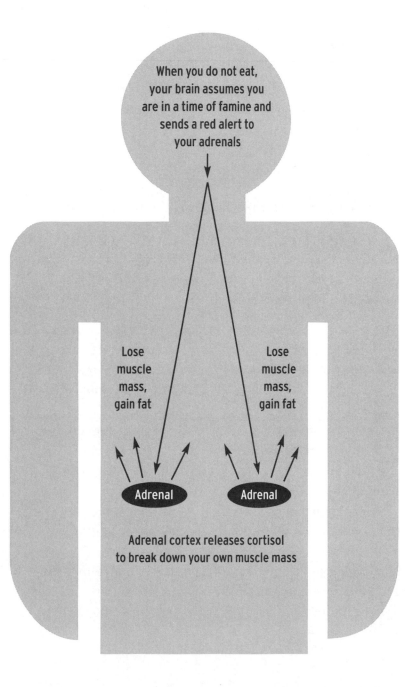

In addition to lacking building blocks of repair and rejuvenation, these foods are acid forming. While it is appropriate and necessary to be in a sympathetic state part of the time, eating processed, junk, or fake foods keeps your body in an acidic state of sympathetic nervous system dominance.

This causes your adrenals to work overtime, which ultimately depletes adrenal reserve. The end result of eating these products is fat around your middle, a flabby body, and accelerated aging. Examples follow some—but not all—of the processed, junk, and fake foods you should avoid.

Food products that keep you in an acidic state of sympathetic dominance

PROCESSED FOOD is made from real food that has been put through devitalizing chemical processes and is infused with chemicals and preservatives:

Beef jerky

Bologna

Cake, brownie, and cookie mixes

Canned foods containing chemicals

Canned or bottled tea and coffee drinks

Canned or jarred gravy and sauces containing chemicals

Canned soup containing chemicals

Hot dogs

Instant cereals and other instant foods

Jams, jellies, preserves, or marmalade with added sugar and chemicals

Low-fat yogurt with sugar or aspartame

Meats containing nitrates

Nuts and seeds roasted in hydrogenated oils

Pasta, bagels, pretzels, pizza, most breads, croissants, muffins, scones

Popcorn popped in hydrogenated oil

Potato chips

Tortilla chips processed in   TV dinners
   hydrogenated oils   White sugar

JUNK FOODS contain very little real food—they are made of devitalized processed food, hydrogenated fats, chemicals, and preservatives:

Anything made with refined   Powdered pudding mixes and
   white flour   pudding snacks
Candy   Sodas, especially those con-
Canned breakfast drinks   taining caffeine and sugar
Cereals (cold, sugary)   substitutes
Doughnuts   Some ice cream products
Drive-through foods   Store-bought cookies
Fried food   Sugary snack foods
"Low calorie" foods   Syrups—fudge, corn, high-
"Low-fat" foods   fructose corn syrup
Pork skins   Toaster pastries

FAKE FOODS are made primarily of chemicals and often contain gums and sugar fillers:

Aspartame   Hydrogenated oils
Bacon bits   Instant coffee
Barbecue sauces   Instant meals—liquid break-
Bottled salad dressing, espe-   fasts, dried noodle soups
   cially diet dressings   Ketchup
Bouillon   Margarine
Butter spreads (imitation)   Marshmallow cream
Cheese (imitation)   Mayonnaise (imitation)
Dehydrated soups   Meat extender
Egg substitutes   Meat tenderizer
Flavor enhancers   Microwaveable and other
Hoisin sauce   imitation food snacks

Non-dairy creamers	Relishes
Oyster sauce	Saccharin
Packaged food helpers	Sandwich spreads
Powdered fruit drinks	Shortening
Powdered, canned, or bottled	Sour cream (imitation)
mixes for making alcoholic	Whipped cream (artificial)
drinks	Worcestershire sauce

I find food journals to be a useful tool. People often surprise themselves when they honestly write down what they eat every day. If you are interested in knowing how much processed, junk, or fake food you eat, keep a journal for one week. Write down everything you eat or drink. You may photocopy these pages or write in a journal.

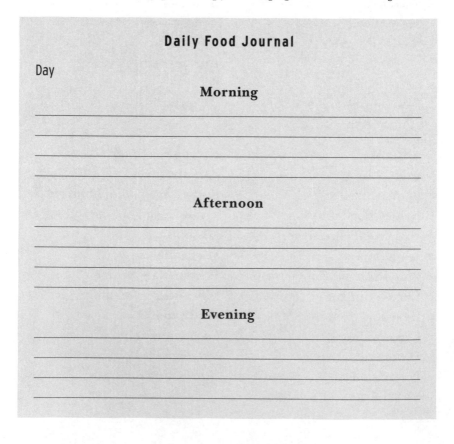

Daily Food Journal

Day

Morning

_____

_____

_____

_____

Afternoon

_____

_____

_____

_____

Evening

_____

_____

_____

_____

Balancing Your Blood Sugar Is in Your Control

I would like you to look at feeding yourself in a completely different light. When it comes to the stress of our modern life, eating is one factor that is in your control. In fact, if you looked at all the factors that contribute to health and well-being as a hierarchy, eating well would be the number one factor. When you eat regular balanced meals of real, whole foods, your blood sugar remains balanced. Think of how wonderful it is that there is something so simple that you are actually in control of—and something you can do for your health that makes such a huge difference.

The purpose of eating is to provide the body with the necessary building materials for ongoing repair, rebuilding, and metabolic processes. The ideal diet is comprised of real whole foods—protein, fat, a small amount of complex carbohydrate, and a nonstarchy vegetable at each meal. When you eat, two hormones, glucagon and insulin, are released from your pancreas. When you eat a balanced diet, these hormones are balanced. Glucagon is responsible for releasing sugar, fat, and proteins from your cells to be used as fuel and building blocks within your body. Insulin is the fat- and nutrient-storing hormone that ushers nutrients into your cells. The ratio between these two hormones determines whether the food you eat will be used as building materials or fuel or stored as fat. A low ratio (higher glucagon) means that a food is likely to be used as building materials or fuel. A high ratio (higher insulin) means that a food is likely to be stored as fat.

Glucagon is released when you eat protein. Insulin is released when you eat sugar (carbohydrates). If you eat only carbohydrates, your insulin-to-glucagon ratio will be too high. If you eat only proteins, your insulin-to-glucagon ratio will be too low.

The insulin-to-glucagon ratio is also determined by the glycemic index of foods, which is a measure of how quickly insulin is released in response to the quantity of sugar entering your system. Simple sugars such as white sugar, honey, pasta, white rice, and processed cereal arrive faster than complex sugars such as yams, potatoes, corn, and brown rice; therefore simple sugars have a higher glycemic index than complex carbohydrates.

Eating a balanced diet of proteins, fats, nonstarchy vegetables—
which provide vitamins, minerals, and fiber—with carbohydrates will
insure a balanced insulin-to-glucagon ratio and a balanced glycemic
index. To make it simple, the following lists are a guide to low, medium,
and high glycemic index foods.

Low glycemic index foods

Proteins (meat, fish, fowl,
eggs, cheese)

Fats and oils (olive oil and
other liquid oils, butter,
cream, sour cream, cheese,
cottage cheese)

Nonstarchy vegetables
(green leafy vegetables
and other low-carbohydrate
vegetables)

Medium glycemic index foods

Beans and legumes

Fruits

Nuts

Starchy vegetables (corn and
tubers)

Whole grains (barley, buck-
wheat, bulgur, millet,
quinoa, rye, wheat, wheat
bran, wheat germ, brown
rice, wild rice)

High glycemic index foods

Flour products

Sugar

Processed, junk, and fake
food

Eating a Balanced Diet of Real, Whole Food

Anyone who regularly skips meals, restricts food intake, or eats a diet
of processed, junk, or fake food will see a dramatic improvement in
overall health and vitality, an immediate drop in body fat, and a star-
tling shift in body composition by simply switching to a diet of real,

whole food. Real food is anything that you could theoretically pick, gather, milk, hunt, or fish—foods that are very close to a natural state.

Real foods

Dairy products such as eggs, butter, cream, milk, and cheese	Nuts
	Oils, especially essential fatty acids (seed, nut, and fish oils)
Fish and shellfish	
Fruits	Poultry
Grains	Sea algae (green food)
Legumes	Seeds
Meat	Vegetables

Eating is the first Simple Solution because just balancing your blood sugar by eating properly will take the majority of demand off your adrenals—even if you cannot make any other changes. If the idea of eating seems too complicated or inconvenient, look again at your psychogene and try to understand why you resist feeding yourself. Chrisy believed that there was safety in perfection, and her fear of imperfection → led to anxiety, nerves, and jitters → led to blindly driving herself → led to nervous breakdown and bankruptcy. In this equation Chrisy was so busy making sure her exterior world was perfect that she had no time to take care of herself.

Your psychogene may be telling you that you are too busy with other more important details to prepare and eat meals. The fact is that nourishing your body will give you more of an edge to be successful than any other factor. When you feel and look healthy and vital, you will have more stamina, a more optimistic attitude about life, greater ability to deal with life's issues, and more self-confidence.

**When you consistently eat balanced meals
of real, whole foods you will**

Lose weight

Increase your metabolism

Burn away fat around your
   middle

Develop ideal body
   composition

Have less cellulite

If you are in the Driven or Dragging stages, three balanced meals of real, whole foods a day will keep your blood sugar levels balanced and will fire up your metabolism. If you are in the Losing It, Hitting the Wall, or especially the Burned Out stage, to restore adrenal function and to fire up your metabolism you need to eat five times a day— I call it grazing. If you are suffering from insomnia, add a bedtime snack. Eat six times a day so as to have the same amount of food as in three good meals spread out over the entire day. Begin each day with a balanced breakfast as soon as possible after awakening, even if it is a small snack. Power drinks are great beginnings—especially if you find food unappealing in the morning. You will find recipes for power drinks on pages 334–339 in chapter 15. These drinks are made of essential fatty acids, fiber, protein, and nutrient foods that will help your adrenals repair. In addition to adding power drinks, begin to eat every two to three hours. Grazing will keep your blood sugar levels balanced and in so doing will allow your adrenals to Rest, Repair, and Rejuvenate. This will expedite your adrenals' healing process—even if you cannot make larger changes such as exercise or changing to a less stressful job.

If you are in the Losing It, Hitting the Wall, or Burned Out stage and are eating six times a day, once you have established a better overall balance in your eating habits—and your adrenals have repaired and replenished their reserves—you may not need to eat quite so often. There is no set timeframe, and everyone is different. Your body will let you know when your adrenals have repaired and replenished their reserves.

Some signs of adrenal repair

Your body has reached its ideal composition—your body mass has shifted to more muscle and less fat

Your cravings have ended

Your moods have evened out

You are sleeping soundly

You feel healthier and more vital than you have in years

You feel an increased sense of self-confidence and creativity

Losing Weight

Sixty-year-old Richard Kantor had been in the fashion industry for forty years. The fashion world seems to have a special patina all its own, but to Richard it meant stress, deadlines, uncertainty, and skipping meals. At six feet tall, Richard was thirty-five pounds overweight. He seemed depressed, and as we talked I found that he was feeling down and stressed out. "The fashion industry is built on artificial deadlines," Richard explained. "If you don't meet the deadlines, you lose orders and a tremendous amount of money. You have to deliver by a given date, and if you don't, stores can cancel the order, and you're sitting there with a lot of clothing. There's a tremendous amount of stress in clothing manufacturing, and there is absolutely no respite. I have been doing it for forty years. It's not easy to deflect the stress, and over the years it has started to wear on me and my body."

The All-Protein, No-Carbohydrate Diet

Richard, who had been highly ambitious and stressed out for four decades, was ready to make some changes. He wanted to lose weight and asked me about cutting carbohydrates. There is much controversy today about how many carbohydrates to eat per meal. Many people are eliminating carbohydrates altogether from their diets— which is not wise. Your body functions optimally on a balanced diet.

There are a number of reasons not to go on an all-protein, no-carbohydrate diet.

- Going without a basic food group is another way to imbalance your blood sugar.

- Most people who go on an all-protein diet eat primarily animal proteins. Animal proteins contain an abundance of a fatty acid called Omega 6. Although some Omega 6 is important for good health, excess Omega 6 blocks the absorption of another important fatty acid called Omega 3. Omega 3 is essential for life. Too much Omega 6 and not enough Omega 3 has been shown to be a major contributing factor in the development of cancer. The right amount of Omega 6 can be obtained by eating a balanced diet.

- Since the release of the good mood neurotransmitter serotonin is stimulated by eating carbohydrates, eliminating them from your diet can sink you into a deep depression.

- Proteins such as meat, fish, shellfish, fowl, eggs, and dairy products provide the building blocks for muscle mass, hormones, and neurotransmitters and the repair, rebuilding, and metabolic processes within your body. They are also acid-forming foods, so you do not want to eat them without eating alkalizing foods such as complex carbohydrates and nonstarchy vegetables.

What Is the Right Amount of Carbohydrates to Eat?

When people think of nutrition they immediately think of weight loss. Instead of making losing weight your goal, focus on eating balanced meals of real, whole foods that will even out your blood sugar. When your blood sugar levels remained balanced, your adrenals can build backup reserves. Your brain will not tell your adrenals to pump adrenaline and cortisol into your body to release sugar any more. Your system will function more efficiently, and your body will gradually become capable of building muscle and burning fat. Your weight will naturally seek a healthy plateau, and your ideal body will emerge.

Carbohydrates turn into sugar in your body, which is used as fuel. Carbohydrates do not make muscle and bones, hormones, or neurotransmitters—these are made from proteins and fats. To stay healthy and to have an ideal body composition, carbohydrates are the one food group for which you need to pay attention to portion control.

Healthy weight loss means that you are losing fat. If your goal is to lose body fat and you are losing more than two pounds per week, no matter how thrilling it is to get on the scale, you are in a self-defeating mode—because this weight is muscle mass, not fat. As you lose muscle mass, your metabolism is lowered, and there will be a backlash of weight gain sooner or later. If you are losing weight too fast, increase your complex carbohydrate consumption slightly until your weight loss slows down to no more than two pounds a week.

The recommendations that follow are provided to help you begin to eat meals and snacks of proteins, fats, and nonstarchy vegetables with a portion of complex carbohydrates. Allow yourself to be flexible with these guidelines. See page 363 for where you can find a complete carbohydrate counter.

Animal proteins and fats do not contain carbohydrates. Nonstarchy vegetables such as green leafy vegetables contain negligible amounts of carbohydrates. Nuts and seeds, fruit, starchy vegetables, legumes, grains, milk, and yogurt all contain carbohydrates.

To understand how many carbohydrates you are likely to need per meal, begin by determining how active you are.

Couch Potato

You drive to work, take the elevator instead of taking the stairs, and sit at a desk. At night and weekends you find yourself lounging in front of the TV. There are times, such as family outings to the beach or company picnics, when you could swim or play softball, but you generally beg off and avoid exertion. I recommend that Couch Potatoes begin with 15 grams of carbohydrate per meal and 10 grams per snack. When you reach your ideal weight, or if you lose weight too fast or feel lethargic or depressed on this amount of carbohydrate, increase to 30 grams of carbohydrate per meal and 15 grams of carbohydrate per snack.

Active at Work

You are a nurse, grade school teacher, or flight attendant or have a similarly active occupation that keeps you moving, bending, and walking all day. Begin with 25 grams of carbohydrate per meal and 15 grams per snack. When you reach your ideal weight, or if you lose weight too fast or feel lethargic or depressed on this amount of carbohydrate, increase to 30 grams of carbohydrate per meal and 15 grams of carbohydrate per snack.

Active Lifestyle

You enjoy two to four hours a week of sports such as shooting baskets, beach walking, yoga, or golf. Begin with 25 to 30 grams of carbohydrate per meal and 15 to 20 grams per snack. When you reach your ideal weight, or if you lose weight too fast or feel lethargic or depressed on this amount of carbohydrate, increase to 30 to 40 grams of carbohydrate per meal and 15 to 20 grams of carbohydrate per snack.

Athletic

Exercise is up there on your list of priorities, and although you may not have time to exercise every day, your total exercise equals at least seven hours a week of moderately challenging sports such as biking, aerobics, power yoga, skiing, jogging, or weight training. Or you have a physically demanding job such as a package delivery or a baggage handling. Begin with 30 to 45 grams of carbohydrate per meal and 20 to 25 grams per snack. When you reach your ideal weight, or if you lose weight too fast or feel lethargic or depressed on this amount of carbohydrate, increase to 50 to 60 grams of carbohydrate per meal and 30 grams of carbohydrate per snack.

Diehard

You hit the track for two hours a day and then lift weights for an hour. You go for extreme sports such as long distance biking, ashtanga yoga, rock climbing, marathons and iron man competitions, competitive swimming, and body building. Begin with 45 to 70 grams of carbohydrate per meal and 35 grams per snack. When you reach your ideal weight, or if you lose weight too fast or feel lethargic or depressed on this amount of carbohydrate, increase to 80 grams of carbohydrate per meal and 60 grams of carbohydrate per snack.

When Richard first walked into my office he was Hitting the Wall. I now consider Richard my poster boy for recovering from adrenal burnout—and living proof that you can regain your health, vitality, and optimistic attitude about life. He also proved that you can change your body composition at any age. Richard regained the musculature of a much younger man and was able to enjoy hours of roller-skating, weight lifting, and bicycling. He was happy to be alive and ready to take on new challenges and a completely different career instead of fading into retirement. "In three and a half months of eating a balanced diet, thirty-eight pounds just melted off my body," Richard said. "My face got younger. I'm like a kid, I have so much energy."

Overweight individuals have a lot of potential energy to burn. If you are overweight, by balancing your meals, cutting out processed foods and sugar, and putting the emphasis on being healthy rather than seeing your weight drop on the scale, you will lose body fat. All of a sudden your body will be able to access the energy you have been storing as fat and you will have a ton of energy.

The End of the Low-fat, Low-cholesterol Diet

A key factor in Richard's remarkable recovery was the addition of cholesterol to his diet. He added two eggs for breakfast every morning. Eating cholesterol, in foods such as eggs, has been long thought to be the cause of heart disease. The so-called lipid hypothesis promoted the belief that elevated blood cholesterol levels were a risk factor for heart disease—and that blood cholesterol levels were elevated by eating cholesterol-laden foods. Mary Enig, Ph.D, is an internationally recognized biochemist in the field of fats and oils and an authority on transfatty acids. For many years Dr. Enig was one of the lone voices speaking out against the lipid hypothesis, and she has dedicated over two decades of research to disproving this theory. In an interview for this book Dr. Enig said: "Eating cholesterol is essential for life. Cholesterol is the body's repair substance. Cholesterol maintains the integrity of cells and membranes. It is used and needed by every cell in your body and is the precursor to all sex hormones. It is needed for proper brain function. The older you are the more you need to eat cholesterol for your cognitive function.

"The lipid hypothesis has been disproven in many scientific studies. In fact, it has been shown that blood cholesterol levels are not a risk factor for heart disease. Furthermore, it has been shown that eating cholesterol raises cholesterol in individuals whose cholesterol is too low and lowers cholesterol levels in individuals whose cholesterol is too high. The egg industry was naturally very interested in this subject and has recently published the results of a large study that demonstrates that eating eggs actually lowers cholesterol."

Richard commented, "I had high cholesterol, but I started eating fourteen eggs a week and my cholesterol dropped like a stone. My cholesterol dropped from two hundred eighty to two twenty. My triglycerides were two hundred and ninety and they dropped to forty-seven." Not everyone will have the same results as Richard. The goal is to eat a balanced diet.

The End of the Low-fat Diet

Your body uses naturally occurring oils for numerous processes such as building all of your cell membranes—including those of your brain, tissues, and organs—and making enzymes, neurotransmitters, and hormones. Finally, more doctors and the public are becoming aware that the low-fat diet fad of the 1980s and 1990s is not the way to health and balance. Eating a low-fat diet is a surefire way to put your adrenals into red alert that your body is in a dangerous famine. It is the way to *increase* body fat, malnutrition, and risk of heart attacks and chronic disease and is clearly a major stressor for your body.

What a low-fat diet will do for you

Brittle nails and dry thinning hair

Chronic degenerative diseases such as osteoarthritis, coronary artery disease, high blood pressure, osteoporosis, stroke, and type II diabetes

Constipation

Cravings for sugar and stimulants

Dry, itchy, scaly skin, including cracked fingers and heels

Fat around the middle and an overall flabby body

Infertility

Insomnia and extreme fatigue

Malnutrition

Mood swings, depression, and other emotional disorders

Healthy Fats Can Help End Cravings

One of the most disturbing problems of our age is eating disorders, cravings for food, and out-of-control eating. According to Dr. Enig, "Animal foods containing saturated fat and cholesterol provide vital nutrients necessary for growth, energy, and protection from degenerative disease. Animal fats are necessary for reproduction. Humans are drawn to both by powerful instincts. Suppression of natural appetites, such as eating processed fats instead of natural fats, leads to weird nocturnal habits, fantasies, fetishes, bingeing, and splurging."

You can end cravings and overeating by eating a balanced diet of real, whole foods, including good fats. Think of your metabolism as a campfire. The carbohydrates you eat are the kindling—they flame up fast but burn quickly away. Proteins are the larger branches that burn longer. Fats are the logs that burn for hours and hours—keeping your metabolism fired up. Eating good fats can actually spark your metabolism and fat-burning processes. You will lose weight and have more energy.

In addition to following a balanced diet, using a weight loss formula that contains healthy fatty acids can speed up your metabolism and help to burn off fat. This formula will not cause you to lose weight if you are at a healthy weight. It will act as a regulator—if you are overweight, you can lose weight until you reach your optimal body composition. Of course, it is also important to eat a balanced diet of real, whole foods, including proteins, fats, a little bit of carbohydrate, and vegetables. You do not need doctor supervision to use this formula, and you can take it along with your other supplements.

Losing Weight

Weight Loss Formula

Take 30 to 60 minutes before each meal:

- 25 milligrams thiamin (vitamin B1)
- 10 milligrams riboflavin (vitamin B2)
- 25 milligrams niacin
- 70 milligrams magnesium
- 5 milligrams zinc
- 200 micrograms chromium
- 5 milligrams vanadium
- *Also add:* 500 milligrams conjugated linoleic acid and 20 milligrams rosemary leaf extract

Saturated Fats

You have heard the terms *saturated, polyunsaturated,* and *monounsaturated,* but perhaps you do not really understand the difference. These fatty acids differ from each other in molecular structure.

Research has been going on for the last fifty years that demonstrates that eating meat, butter, eggs, and cream does *not* contribute to heart disease. The food industry—which thrives on the sales of fake foods such as egg substitutes and margarine—has succeeded in brainwashing the public and suppressing these findings. For decades we all believed that these natural foods were harmful. "The truth is that we are better off eating the real food that human beings have always lived on," said Dr. Enig. "Saturated fats are part of a balanced diet. The human body functions best when it has good quality raw materials, such as saturated fats." It makes common sense that the human body would thrive on a real, organic egg and not have a clue what to do with a chemical-laden imitation egg product.

We have all heard it said that we eat too much fat and that fat consumption has risen since the turn of the twentieth century. Statistics prove this to be false. Fat consumption has not changed at all. What has changed is the types of fats people eat. One hundred years ago people ate naturally occurring fats and oils such as butter, chicken fat, coconut oil, lard, olive oil, and tallow, which are fats from beef and lamb. Today people eat the majority of their fats in manmade hydrogenated fats, such as margarine, and other manmade polyunsaturated oils such as corn oil. Hydrogenated fats have been clearly linked to heart disease and cancer.

What saturated fats do for you

Enhance your immune system
Build healthy bones
Protect your liver
Provide energy and structural
    integrity to your cells

Satisfy you so that you do
    not crave unhealthy
    foods
Stabilize cholesterol levels

Saturated fats are referred to as stable fatty acids. This means that their molecules are not as easily altered by heating. For cooking,

saturated fats are best. There is a complete listing of healthy and unhealthy fats on pages 340–343.

Healthy saturated fats to eat at room temperature or to cook with

Butter	Cream	Palm kernel oil
Cheese	Eggs	Shea nut oil
Cocoa butter	Nutmeg oil	Sour cream
Coconut butter or oil		

One fantastic saturated fat that is just now getting the attention it
deserves is coconut oil. Coconut oil contains lauric acid, which is con-
verted by the body into monolaurin, which is believed to cause the
disintegration of viruses, including HIV, measles, herpes simplex
virus, cytomegalovirus (a serious infectious disease that can cause
mental retardation and death), influenza virus, and pneumonovirus.
Research suggests that the average adult would benefit from 24
grams of lauric acid daily, which can be obtained by eating ½ tablespoon of coconut oil, 10 ounces of pure coconut milk, or 7 ounces of
raw coconut daily. Since allergies to coconut are caused by the proteins, the oil is safe for those who are allergic. You can easily incorporate coconut into your life by making curries, putting coconut milk
into your protein drinks, using coconut butter to cook, and in place
of butter.

Monounsaturated Oils

With the false vilification of saturated fats and the focus on processed
polyunsaturated fats, monounsaturated fats have not gotten the attention they deserve. Since the monounsaturated molecule is not easily damaged, monounsaturated oil can be used for cooking and is
now being used by health-minded manufacturers in cookies and

chips. Always buy oils and products that are labeled pure-, expeller-, or cold-pressed. Because monounsaturated oils are susceptible to damage by oxidation when exposed to light and air, purchase oils packaged in dark bottles whenever possible.

Two of the most popular oils today are safflower and sunflower oils. Depending on where the safflower and sunflower seeds were grown, these oils can have either a monounsaturated or a polyunsaturated composition. Monounsaturated cold-, pure-, or expeller-pressed sunflower and safflower oils are healthy to eat because they have not been damaged by the process that extracted the oil from the seed. These oils are also suitable for cooking, since the monounsaturated oil molecule is relatively stable—and so they are included on the list of healthy oils. It is best to avoid polyunsaturated sunflower and safflower oils, since they are likely to have been processed out of the seeds using high temperatures and are further damaged if you use them for cooking. But since manufacturers have not yet begun to label bottles of sunflower and/or safflower oils as mono- or polyunsaturated, it is best to avoid these two oils until such time as manufacturers make the distinction. However, you will now find more products such as cookies and chips that are labeled as being made with cold-, pure-, or expeller-pressed monounsaturated oil that are healthy to eat.

Healthy monounsaturated fats to eat at room temperature

Almond oil	Grape seed oil	Oat oil
Apricot kernel oil	Hazelnut oil	Rice bran oil
Avocado oil	Mustard oil	Sesame oil
Black currant oil		

Healthy monounsaturated fats to cook with

Chicken fat	Safflower oil if it	Sunflower oil if it is
Duck fat	is cold-, pure-,	cold-, pure-, or
Goose fat	or expeller-	expeller-pressed
Olive oil	pressed	Turkey fat

Polyunsaturated Oils

For many years we have heard that polyunsaturated oil (such as corn oil) is the healthiest oil and that polyunsaturated oils prevented heart disease. It is true that naturally occurring polyunsaturated fats are healthy. Unfortunately, polyunsaturated oil is the least stable oil molecule, which means it is easily damaged by heat. The polyunsaturated oils that have been promoted are oils that have been subjected to damaging industrial processes that have rendered them toxic to the human body.

Fat molecules naturally occur in what is called the "cis molecular configuration." In this configuration, the hydrogen atoms are on the same side of the carbon double bond molecule. The hydrogen atoms repel one another causing the fatty chain to kink up. This bent shape determines the fatty acid molecule's behavior and function in our bodies. In very simple terms, the cis configuration is the natural and healthy molecular configuration that the human body recognizes and is able to use in creating new cells. However, using heat and chemical processes to extract fat from its natural state—such as extracting corn oil from corn—changes the natural cis configuration to a "trans molecular configuration." In the trans configuration, the hydrogen atoms are on opposite sides of the molecule and the molecule straightens out. This trans molecular structure, referred to as a transfatty acid, has never before been incorporated into human physiology and is unrecognizable to the human body. Transfatty acids damage cells and lead to heart disease, cancer, and other degenera-

Figure 5
Cis and trans molecular structures of damaged fats

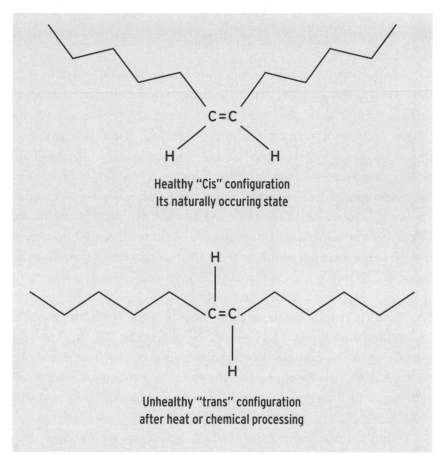

Healthy "Cis" configuration
Its naturally occuring state

Unhealthy "trans" configuration
after heat or chemical processing

tive diseases. Again, the best example of a polyunsaturated transfatty acid is corn oil. Other examples are cottonseed, canola, and shortening—made from vegetable oil.

The generation of transfatty acids also produces free radicals. Free radicals damage cells, which are more likely to mutate into cancer. Free radicals also lead to arthritis, autoimmune disease, premature aging, and heart disease.

We have been told for decades that polyunsaturated fats were good for us—and that saturated fats caused heart disease and cancer. We now know that the opposite is true. Most vegetable oils are toxic when heated. If you heat a cooking pot of heat-processed polyunsaturated oil that is already swimming with transfatty acids and cook French fries in this oil, this creates many more transfatty acid/free radical molecules. When you eat these fries you are now swimming in free radicals.

Another damaging process to polyunsaturated oil is hydrogenation. Hydrogenated and partially hydrogenated fats were developed as a cheap alternative to butter. For example, margarine is made by first extracting oil from corn at a very high heat. Then this damaged polyunsaturated oil is put through a hydrogenation process. This process transforms oil molecules into straight "packable" molecules by rearranging the hydrogen atoms—so that liquid oils can be "packed" into solids. Hydrogenated fats have no health benefits. In fact, fats such as margarine and other fake butter spreads have never before been incorporated into the cellular structure of the human body.

The membranes of all living cells are made of up to 70 percent fat. For a cell to do its job properly, what it absorbs has to be made of the right building blocks—including healthy fat. Just as you would not put sewing machine oil into your car, you should not put damaged oils or hydrogenated fats, which are transfatty acids/free radicals, into the human body. This is what causes obesity and disease.

When you eat transfatty acids, hydrogenated or partially hydrogenated fats, and oxidized fats you end up with rigid cells instead of moist and fluid cells that are functioning well. Rigid cells trap cellular waste, which suffocates cells and causes the failure of internal enzyme systems. The combined result is a breeding ground for diseases such as cancers, chronic inflammatory disease, and autoimmune diseases. The human brain, which is 70 percent fat, has become increasingly composed of damaged fat molecules over the last fifty years. When the cell membranes of the brain cannot communicate properly because they are made of the wrong molecules, we begin to see problems with mental functioning such as autism, ADD, ADHD, Parkinson's, Alzheimer's, and depression.

What hydrogenated and partially hydrogenated fats do to you

Accelerate aging

Compromise the integrity of the immune system

Contribute to risk for developing cancer, heart disease, and type II diabetes

Damage the reproductive organs and lungs

Decrease testosterone in men, increase level of abnormal sperm

Have been linked to mental decline and chromosomal damage

Increase body fat

Increase problems with mental functioning such as autism, ADD, ADHD, Parkinson's disease, Alzheimer's disease, and depression

Increase risk for arthritis and autoimmune disease

Inhibit fertility in women

Create toxicity in the liver

Never eat:

Heat-processed poly- and monounsaturated oils containing transfatty acids

Canola, unless it is cold-, pure-, or expeller-pressed

Mayonnaise made with heat-processed canola oil

Corn oil

Cottonseed oil

Peanut oil—healthy to eat on occasion if it is cold-, pure-, or expeller-pressed

Safflower oil, unless it is cold-, pure-, or expeller-pressed and mono-unsaturated

Sunflower oil, unless it is cold-, pure-, or expeller-pressed and mono-unsaturated

Soy oil

Avoid sources of hydrogenated fats, partially hydrogenated fats, and damaged polyunsaturated oils

Bottled salad dressings	Imitation mayonnaise	Non-dairy creamers
Chips	Imitation sour cream	Pressurized whipped cream
Cookies	Margarine and other hydro-genated fake butter spreads	Processed, junk, and fake foods
Corn oil		Sandwich spreads
Cottonseed oil		Shortening
Deep-fat fried foods		

Healthy Polyunsaturated Oils

Polyunsaturated oils are found in foods such as almonds, salmon, and walnuts. When eaten in their natural state, these oils are fabulously healthy for you. They are also healthy when they are processed out of their natural state by using pure-, cold-, and expeller press techniques, rather than heat-damaging manufacturing processes.

Eating healthy polyunsaturated oil

Slows down accelerated aging
Strengthens your immune system
Lowers your risk for developing cancer, heart disease, and type II diabetes
Supports your reproductive organs and lungs
Decreases body fat
Decreases your risk for arthritis and autoimmune disease
Promotes fertility in women
Decreases ADD, ADHD, Parkinson's disease, Alzheimer's disease, and depression
Is healthy for your liver

Cold-, pure-, or expeller-pressed polyunsaturated essential fatty acids to eat at room temperature

Almond oil	Borage oil	Salmon oil
Apricot oil	Herring oil	Sardine oil
Poppyseed oil	Menhaden (fish)	Walnut oil
Primrose oil	oil	Wheat germ
Flaxseed oil	Sesame seed oil	oil

Omega 3 and Omega 6 Oils

Omega 3 and Omega 6 are in two distinct families of polyunsaturated fatty acids that are vital to many of your body's processes. Omega 3 and 6 fatty acids are essential for life, which is why they are called essential fatty acids.

What Omega 3 oils do for you

Act as a natural antiinflammatory agent
Are a precursor for hormone production—essential for life
Regulate metabolism
Stimulate fat burning

What happens when you do not get Omega 3 oils

Brain dysfunction	Increased behavior disorders
Increased inflammation	Decrease in cognitive ability
Increased chronic illness	

Fish oils are one of the best sources of Omega 3. It is thought that the essential fatty acids in fish tissues and blood helps fishes' membranes to remain fluid instead of turning solid in their cold water environment. The colder the water the fish comes from, the more essential fatty acids the fish contains. Taking salmon oil and deep-sea fish oils in capsule form is a wonderful way to supply your body with nourishing, moisturizing antitumor and antiinflammatory essential fatty acids. Three other oils that provide Omega 3 are hemp, flax, and pumpkin seed oil. Hemp seed oil is the best balanced source of Omega 3 and 6. Hemp seed oil is extracted from *Cannabis sativa,* which is the seed from which marijuana grows. Hemp seeds do not contain THC, which is the primary intoxicant in marijuana and hashish. If you eat hemp oil, it is important to know that there is a chance that drug tests can show positive. Flax and pumpkin seed are the next two best balanced oils.

Although we are deficient in Omega 3, there is far too much Omega 6 in the Western diet of processed foods. An excess of Omega 6 results in more cancers. One of the arguments against eating animal products is that, since toxins are fat soluble, herbicides and pesticides are stored in the fatty tissues of animals. Whenever possible, eat organic dairy as well as free range organic meats. Buy lean cuts of

Sources of Omega 3

Blue-green algae	Fish oil	Sardine oil
Chia seeds	Flaxseed oil	Spirulina (sea
Chlorella (sea	Hemp oil	algae)
algae)	Mackerel oil	Tuna fish
Dunalellia (sea	Pumpkin oil	Walnuts and
algae)	Salmon oil	oil

Sources of Omega 6

Butter	Fowl	Safflower oil
Cream	Grape seed oil	Sunflower oil
Eggs	Hemp oil	Turkey
Fish oil	Meat	Walnuts and oil
Flaxseed oil	Pumpkin oil	Wheat germ oil

meat and trim the fat. Omega 6 is necessary, but it is not healthy to overeat any food group.

The Vegetarian Diet

Many people, especially teenagers, are turning toward the vegetarian diet. I am not opposed to anyone choosing this diet. I ate a vegetarian diet for twelve years until I realized that this diet is extremely difficult to maintain in a healthy way. Most people who avoid animal proteins turn to refined carbohydrates. If you want to eat a vegetarian diet, it is essential for your health that you plan and prepare the proper balance of proteins, fats, and a small amount of real, complex carbohydrates.

Unfortunately, the vegetarian diet can be high in carbohydrate—and fattening. Rice and beans make a complete protein. However, 1 cup of brown rice and 1 cup of beans together contain 86 grams of protein—the amount of protein many people need to spread out over an entire day.

If you choose a vegetarian diet, take care to eat tofu, seeds, legumes, nuts, whole grains, and plenty of nonstarchy vegetables every day. Add saturated animal protein sources of Omega 6, such as cheese and eggs, and fats such as butter and cream—as well as sources of Omega 3 proteins and fats such as fish, if you will allow it.

Whether you are a meat eater or a vegetarian, there cannot be a set formula for the amount of fats and oils one needs because we are all different ages and sizes and have varied activity levels. The issue is the quality of fat you eat.

How to Buy and Use Fats and Oils

Another issue with fats and oils is oxidization, which results when healthy fats are exposed to light, air, heat, and other free radicals. In fact, the very best natural oils spoil easily. In nature, the seed or nut that contains the oil protects it from oxygen. Once the seed is cracked or crushed, oxygen can get to the oil. Oxygen binds to the oil molecule's carbon atom, where the hydrogen atom is missing (the double-bonded carbons), and steals an electron from the fat molecule. The fat is now missing an electron, and is a free radical. This is oxidation or, in common terms, rancidity. Oxidation creates free radicals, which damages cells and genes and leads to cancer, arthritis, autoimmune disease, premature aging, and heart disease.

Simple rules for buying and eating oils

- Buy oils in opaque containers or dark glass bottles.

- When you open a bottle of oil, break open a couple of vitamin E capsules and squirt them into the freshly opened bottle—vitamin E is a natural antioxidant for oil.

- Once oil is opened, keep it refrigerated and use it up as quickly as you can.

- Throw away rancid fats—even if they were expensive.

- Avoid eating deep-fried foods.

- Avoid eating processed, junk, or fake foods made with hydrogenated or partially hydrogenated fats.

- Avoid hydrogenated or partially hydrogenated fats such as margarine and imitation butter spreads.

- Now that people are becoming educated about damaged polyunsaturated oils, manufacturers are beginning to turn to monounsaturated cold-, pure-, or expeller-pressed oils. You can now buy cookies, chips, mayonnaise and other foods made with these healthy oils.

Fruits and Vegetables

As your body strives to maintain a narrow pH range, it is helped or hindered by the types of foods you eat. Real foods, such as fruits and vegetables, that are high in minerals, certain alkaline amino acids, and dietary enzymes are essential for the pH regulatory process. It is important to add plenty of vegetables and fruits to your diet. These foods provide vitamins and minerals, but they also contain fiber that attracts toxins and pulls them out of your body before they can be reabsorbed or recycled.

Acid and Alkaline Foods

When prehistoric humans lived in the wild, they chose from fresh fruits and vegetables that helped to alkalinize their bodies as well as provide the building blocks needed to buffer acidity. The processed junk and/or fake foods that we eat too much of are acid forming. The processed, junk, and fake foods listed earlier in this chapter are acid forming.

Not all acid-forming foods are bad for you. Balance is the goal. Meat, fish, shellfish, fowl, eggs, and dairy are acid forming; they also provide the building blocks for muscle mass, hormones, and the neurotransmitters that are the backbone of repair, rebuilding, and metabolic processes within your body. You can neutralize the acid from these foods by eating alkaline-forming foods. When your diet is rich in alkaline-forming foods your body will have a greater resistance to disease. Alkaline-forming foods are also crucial to healing. If you are recovering from cancer or a chronic illness, a 50 to 70 percent alkaline diet will help promote healing. A list of alkalinizing foods appears on pages 347–349.

Power Drinks

The main ingredients in power drinks are super green food, stabilized rice bran, and protein powder.

Super Green Food

A fabulous and easy way to get a daily infusion of nutrients is to drink juices made from nature's most potent, nutrient-dense, and clean foods left on earth, known as super green foods. These famous sea vegetables—chlorella; spirulina; special red, blue, green, and brown algae; and dried sea vegetable powders—all bring a variety of powerful nutrients and antioxidants to your diet. In fact, recent studies have demonstrated that green foods lower free radicals in the body and increase longevity. Green foods are naturally alkaline, so they buffer the body's tendency to become acidic under stress.

There are a number of quality freeze-dried green food products that contain all-natural, synergistically blended powders containing vitamins, minerals, trace minerals, enzymes, essential amino acids, and antioxidants. In addition to green organic grasses, blue-green algae, and sea algae, green food products generally contain various herbs, fiber, and bioflavonoid extracts (another form of antioxidant), as well as probiotics cultures—billions of live organisms that benefit the gastrointestinal tract.

You can mix these powders into a protein drink or take six to ten capsules every day. Green foods complete what is missing in our diet. Products that are blended with a variety of ingredients, rather than straight spirulina, generally have a neutral taste and take on the taste of the ingredients they are mixed into.

Stabilized Rice Bran

Next to super green food, stabilized rice bran is the most powerful, potent, nutrient-packed super food. It is very high in antioxidants and phytonutrients—nutrients that naturally exist in plants. Stabilized rice bran lowers cholesterol. It helps to stabilize blood sugar and has been shown in clinical tests to reduce the need for insulin in diabetics. It is made from the husk of the rice that is usually thrown away when rice is milled. The husk has all the antioxidants, vitamins, and phytonutrients.

Protein Powder

Eating protein powder is a convenient way to boost your daily protein intake. Many people who have no appetite for breakfast find power drinks a great way to start their morning.

Since the release of many studies demonstrating that women in cultures such as Japan and China, who eat a lot of soy foods, have less breast cancer, Americans have begun to eat more soy. Eastern women may have less breast cancer, but it is not only because of eating soy. Soy contains several naturally occurring compounds that are toxic to humans and animals in excess. In fact, it has been shown that when soy is fed exclusively to some growing animals they do not grow properly. Eastern women generally eat soy as pieces of tempeh, miso, and tofu and small amounts of sprouted soybeans or as a condiment such as soy sauce or miso; the fermenting process neutralizes the toxicity of soy. In Japan the main protein sources are primarily fish, chicken, and eggs. In China the main protein sources are duck, pork, chicken, fish, and eggs.

In the United States soy was originally grown on fields and then turned under as a source of nitrogen to the soil so that another crop could grow. Today the soy industry extracts the fat from soybeans and puts it through a hydrogenation process. This hydrogenated soy fat is used in processed products such as cookies and crackers. What is left of the soybean is called soy isolate, which is now being touted as healthy, but it is really not safe to eat in great quantities or as an exclusive protein source because it can block the action of certain enzymes and the absorption of some minerals.

When choosing a protein powder, I recommend an alternative such as cold-processed whey protein—which is a wonderful and powerful immune stimulant. Rice and egg protein powders are also available.

Use products that contain between 15 to 20 grams of protein per serving and preferably not more than 5 grams of carbohydrate. Servings are measured by the scoop that is enclosed in the container by the manufacturer.

You can find super green food, stabilized rice bran, and protein powder at your health food store, or you can order a premixed formula online. See page 355 for product recommendations. Recipes for power drinks can be found on pages 334–339.

Recommended Essential Fatty Acids (EFAs)

Essential fatty acid blends are formulated to provide a healthy daily dose of Omega 3 and 6 oils. The further you have progressed through the stages of burnout, the greater will be your need for EFAs. There are numerous healthy blends of EFAs at your health food store. You will either find them in capsules or bottled and refrigerated. If you are making power drinks, the easiest way to include good EFAs is to add 1 teaspoon to 1 tablespoon to your power drink. If you are not drinking power drinks, two to four capsules a day will provide you with your EFAs.

> Essential Balance by Omega Oils
> Omega Twin by Barleans
> Udo's Choice
> Ultimate Oil by Nature's Secret
> Ultra Oil by Country Life
> Wild Alaskan Salmon Oil by Natural Factors

Meal Plans

Trying to decide what to eat every day sends many people straight to the nearest drive-through. Beginning on page 308, you will find two weeks of balanced meal plans of real, whole foods—and easy-to-make recipes.

If you have been yo-yo dieting for years and your metabolism is extremely low, as with any of the Simple Solutions, make small changes. Weight gain can be discouraging—and that is certainly not the goal. Introduce eating changes slowly, giving your body a chance to understand that the time of famine is over and that it does not have to store everything you eat. In a very short period of time you will be able to eat normally without gaining weight.

These meal plans were designed to help you better understand the variety of foods you can eat in one day. Choose what you like from these menus and make up your own. When you make a stew, you can have it for dinner and for lunch the following day—or even for a snack. It takes practice to get into the habit of preparing meals, but it is worth it, both for the sheer pleasure of eating and for the good health it will bring you.

Making the commitment to eat regular balanced meals of real food is the most important solution for your weary adrenals. Use the following checklist of the foods you need to help you choose the right foods throughout the day:

- Protein

- Fat

- Nonstarchy (green) vegetables

- Complex carbohydrate

- Alkalinizing food

Remember, if you fall between Losing It and Burned Out, or if you are not sleeping well, you will need six small meals per day until you have energy to burn and your sleep is regular and reliable. So eat, eat, eat, back to health and healing.

Simple Solution 1: Eat, Eat, Eat, All Day Long
Tailored to your stage of burnout

Driven and Dragging

___ By skipping meals and eating junk food, you are depleting your adrenal reserves. Eating regular balanced meals of real, whole foods will keep your blood sugar balanced and protect your adrenal glands.

___ Avoid lowering your metabolism by never skipping meals or dieting again.

___ Stop eating the deadly, devitalized processed, junk, and fake foods that will age you.

___ Determine the amount of carbohydrates that are right for you. If you lose more than two pounds per week, increase your complex carbohydrate consumption slightly until your weight loss slows down to no more than two pounds a week.

___ You are probably not suffering from cravings and weight gain yet. If you begin to eat healthy fats and oils, including essential fatty acids, you can prevent cravings from starting.

___ If you want to stay as healthy and vital as you are today, never eat heat-processed or hydrogenated fats—they will damage you on a cellular level.

___ Incorporate alkaline-forming foods into your diet every day.

Losing It

___ You are midway to Burned Out. It is vital that you begin to eat regular balanced meals of real, whole foods to balance your blood sugar and to restore adrenal reserves.

___ Why let your metabolism bottom out? Prevent your metabolism from down-regulating any further by never dieting or skipping meals again.

___ You are what you have eaten all these years. So stop eating deadly, devitalized processed, junk, and fake foods now.

___ To restore adrenal function and to fire up your metabolism, begin to eat five times a day—add a bedtime snack if you are suffering from insomnia.

___ Determine the amount of carbohydrates that is right for you. If you lose more than two pounds per week, increase your complex carbohydrate consumption slightly until your weight loss slows down to no more than two pounds a week.

___ Eating healthy fats and oils, especially essential fatty acids, will help your adrenals heal faster.

___ Why eat processed or hydrogenated fats when your body wants the real thing? Eat butter, olive oil, and other natural fats and oils for improved health and vitality.

___ Make alkaline-forming foods a part of your diet. Make a pact with yourself to eat more vegetables.

Hitting the Wall and Burned Out

___ To save your life you must eat regular balanced meals of real, whole foods. A balanced diet will balance your blood sugar and to begin to restore your ravaged adrenal glands.

___ Now is not the time to think about losing weight. Instead, begin to increase your metabolism by saying good-bye to dieting and skipping meals forever.

___ More than ever, now is the time to avoid deadly, devitalized processed, junk, and fake foods. Your body does not have the reserve to fight off these poisons.

___ It is imperative that you begin to eat six small meals a day. Grazing throughout the day will help restore your adrenal function and heal your metabolism.

___ Determine the amount of carbohydrates that is right for you. If you are losing more than two pounds per week, increase your complex carbohydrate consumption slightly until your weight loss slows down to no more than two pounds a week. You may need a little more carbohydrate at these stages. Never go hungry again.

___ Healthy fats and oils, such as butter, olive oil, and essential fatty acids will provide your body with the raw materials to make new cells.

___ Eating processed and hydrogenated fats would be like throwing gasoline on a fire. Clean out your cupboards and refrigerator now and throw anything away that is made with these damaged fats.

___ Now it is critical to eat alkaline-forming foods at every meal. Every meal should be multicolored with plenty of vegetables.

5

Simple Solution 2
Exercise Less

Less exercise is MORE

Shortcuts to Simple Solution 2

- Exercise less to protect your adrenal reserves and keep your metabolism fired up.

- Regular, moderate exercise, doing what you love will keep you healthy.

- Think positive thoughts about exercise to create healthy neurotransmitters.

Fifty-year-old songwriter Grace Wolczak regularly drives out of town into the Southern California foothills to hike with her dogs. "I don't enjoy working out in gyms," Grace said. "The scene has never interested me, and I can't stand all that clanging noise from the machines and the artificial lighting. I love being outdoors where my thoughts can flow and I can be creative."

Grace was a Diehard jogger for twenty years who learned that prolonged overexercise can result in a lowered metabolism and weight gain. She also learned that exercising less is MORE—that less exercise can actually increase your metabolism and lead to fat burning. Like many longtime Diehards, Grace learned the hard way that there are a number of misconceptions about exercise. Perhaps the greatest of those misconceptions is that exercise has to be hard for it to be beneficial, that if there is no pain, there is no gain. But the truth is that the "no pain, no gain" philosophy has caused some people to burn out. "I was twenty-four when I started jogging in 1974. The first pair of running shoes I bought were men's because they didn't make running shoes for women back then. It wasn't even socially acceptable for women to sweat. People used to look at me funny when I would come in from a long run with sweat running down my legs. I ran six miles a day, 360 days a year, for nearly ten years. Every year, on my birthday I would run ten miles. My life pretty much revolved around running. If I was invited out for the evening, I would think, is it worth staying up late? I liked to go to bed early so I could get up early and run. I loved the solitude and the exhilaration. It's just inexplicable to someone who hasn't experienced the high."

Diehards

Just as there are many misconceptions about exercise, there are many truths too. As Grace said, exercise can be exhilarating. We have all heard about—and some have experienced—the runner's high. Diehards' addiction to exercise is in part an addiction to the release of endorphins and dopamine. Endorphins are internal opiates that reduce the sensation of pain and heighten pleasurable emotions. Dopamine is an excitatory, feel-good neurotransmitter. Addictions are commonly related to raising dopamine levels. Some people raise dopamine levels by using cocaine, marijuana, sugar, cigarettes, and alcohol. Others, like Grace, raise dopamine levels by running. Diehards love the feeling they get when endorphins and dopamine are released in their brains. What they do not understand is that they are getting off on a rush at the expense of their adrenals.

Overexercising is an addiction just like cocaine. Like cocaine, overexercising tears your body down faster than it can repair and re-plenish itself. The extreme demand of overexercising triggers the sympathetic nervous system's fight-or-flight mode. Using running as an example, it is logical that your brain would perceive this activity as a response to danger—why else would you run for a half an hour to two hours or longer?

Overexercising Can Make You Fat

When you engage in an extreme sport, because your brain perceives danger it sends a red alert to your adrenals to release cortisol and DHEA to help keep you alive. Although cortisol breaks down muscle mass, DHEA is right there building it back up. At the same time DHEA burns fat. That is why young people who indulge in extreme sports look fit and muscular.

However, if you overexercise for a prolonged period of time, the excessive demand on your adrenals will cause them to fatigue. "From age twenty-four to age thirty-eight my weight stayed the same—or maybe dipped a little when I was working out more," said Grace. "I started to gain weight right around the time I turned forty. So I began working out and running twice as much. But I couldn't get back to my normal weight." When you persist in overexercising over long pe-riods of time, your fatigued adrenals will not be able to produce enough DHEA. Now when you overexercise you have too much cor-tisol and not enough DHEA. Since cortisol breaks down muscle, with-out the DHEA to build it back up, you will have muscle wasting. Since muscle mass dictates the rate of your metabolism, you will have a low-ered metabolism. With your lowered metabolism and less DHEA to burn fat, you are likely to gain body fat. Now instead of being fit and muscular you will begin to show signs of cellulite and fat around the middle.

In addition to the wear and tear on your adrenals, overexercising takes a toll on your entire body. It has been said that it takes three months for the human body to fully repair itself from a twenty-five-mile marathon. So you can imagine if a person exercises vigorously every day how much repair that person's body needs. This repair cannot occur completely in one night's rest or with one good meal. "By age forty-four I couldn't run every day," Grace said. "I had cartilage deterioration in both knees. Also, I just didn't have any more of the monumental driving energy it takes to get out and pound the road day after day." Some of us have great genes, and we can live on our reserve. But no reserve can last forever. It is like having a trust fund. When you spend the entire principal, there is nothing left to accrue interest. You may think: *my energy has always been there—why is it gone now?*

Overexercising Takes a Toll on Your Entire Body

Overexercising cannot continue indefinitely without taking a toll on your adrenals and your body. Many factors need to be considered. For example, some people eat well, others eat sugar and junk. Some make time for play and rest, others are workaholics who rarely take time off. In addition to individual habits, everyone is born with his or her own particular genetic predisposition and adrenal reserve. (Adrenal reserve does not mean the amount of adrenal hormones your adrenal glands are capable of producing over a lifetime. Adrenal reserve is the capacity of your glands to continue to meet the demand at any and every given moment.) A person who is born with

---

Overexercising can result in

Cartilage degeneration	Sick, achy feeling after
Cravings for sugar, caffeine,	exercise
and other stimulants	Symptoms of hypoglycemia
Fatigue	such as foggy-headedness,
Insomnia	shakiness, irritability, and
Muscle wasting	lack of mental clarity
Premature aging	Weight gain

a healthy adrenal reserve and has good living habits might be able to get away with overexercising for many years. I think it is safe to say that nearly everyone who reaches the age of forty has burned out some amount of their adrenal reserve. Therefore those, like Grace, who overexercise past forty will feel the consequences.

If you are a Diehard, start listening to your body. Fatigue and weight gain are clear messages from your body that you are over- doing it. "Giving up jogging was traumatic," Grace said. "It was a big part of my identity. It's an ego thing. I tried power walking, but I felt like hiding behind a tree when someone jogged by me. When I took up hiking it was a new challenge, but it wasn't the same as jogging. I started practicing yoga then. I still miss jogging, but now, at fifty, I'm doing handstands, headstands, and backbends—things I couldn't even do as a child. So I feel that I have a new challenge, and that is something I thrive on. More important, yoga doesn't deplete me. I can go into a class feeling run-down and come out feeling energized. It's the way I felt twenty-five years ago when I got my second wind."

Grace was surprised that she found an exercise that she liked as much as jogging. There are alternatives to extreme sports that will engender adrenal regeneration that will make you feel better and lose weight, and are likely to make you live longer.

There are exceptions. Overexercising can be beneficial for those, for example, teenagers and young men, who have more energy than can be easily burned off in our sedentary, technological society. Too much energy can be a setup for trouble, whether it is a nuclear reac- tor or a flash flood or a human body. Exercise gives these people a venue for using their energy constructively and pleasurably. But our habits have to change as our bodies change with age.

The polar opposites of Diehards are the Couch Potatoes. This is not to imply that there are only two types of people when it comes to ex- ercise. Like any other factor of good health, there are many shades of gray—and there are many types of exercisers. I am singling out the Diehards and the Couch Potatoes merely because they have the hard- est time making changes.

Couch Potatoes

If you have not been goaded out of your chair by visions of fashion models in magazine articles extolling the virtues of exercise, I am not surprised. It might help inspire you if you understood why regular moderate exercise is critical for life.

Regular Moderate Exercise Will Give You More Energy

When we hold still by sitting in a chair or lying on the couch, we atrophy. In fact, after only three days in bed people start to lose muscle. Since muscle mass burns the most energy, when we lose muscle we burn less energy and store more fat. Many years ago a friend made a needlepoint for me that says: "Use it or lose it." It says the truth so beautifully. When we hold still, we start to disintegrate.

For many, exercise is a great solution for fatigue. Most of us have more pent-up energy than we realize, and that energy must move for our bodies to recharge. A battery's charge is the separation of the positive and the negative. When a battery loses its charge, or runs down, it means that the positive and the negative are no longer separated. Think of your body as a battery. When you hold still too long the charge weakens and eventually becomes neutral. When you are physically active, the internal electromagnetic battery of your body is actively recharged.

Regular Moderate Exercise Will Help You Lose Weight and Live Longer

Being overweight has been shown to shorten your life. On the other hand, physically fit people are more apt to live longer. If you are interested in losing body fat and feeling more energetic, less exercise is MORE.

In a healthy individual who eats a regular balanced diet, moderate exercise for longer periods of time causes fat burning. When you first begin to exercise, your adrenal glands produce adrenaline, which raises your heart rate and directs the blood flow to the muscles that are working. Adrenaline also releases blood sugar into your bloodstream to generate the initial energy to fuel your muscles. As you continue to exercise moderately, the hormone glucagon is released from your pancreas. Glucagon is the fat-utilizing hormone. During moderate exercise, glucagon releases fat from your fat cells to turn into sugar to burn as fuel. Since your body has sugar to burn, it means that your brain does not have to call on your adrenals to release cortisol to regulate your blood sugar. At the same time, DHEA is continually released the entire time you are exercising. DHEA also stimulates your body to burn fat for fuel. Switching into fat-burning metabolism releases energy. You will lose body fat and feel more energetic. If you increase the intensity of your exercise without gradual training, your body will switch into alarm mode and you will not have glucagon production, but you will have increased cortisol. As you know by now, high cortisol leads to muscle wasting, lowered metabolism, and weight gain. The better trained you are, the further you can go without getting into cortisol production—that is an important aspect of athletic training.

It is important to note that your body needs a regular supply of protein for glucagon production. When you do not eat sufficient protein, your glucagon production will decline. Then when you exercise, your brain will be forced to call on cortisol to release blood sugar from your muscles for energy. No fat will be burned.

As we age, our bodies repair more slowly and less effectively. Regular moderate exercise slows the aging process and prolongs your life. When we exercise moderately we stimulate the release of human growth hormone (hGH) from the pituitary, which helps activate all the metabolic and repair systems in our body. HGH is the most potent longevity hormone known. HGH accelerates repair of all tissues, stimulates immunity, increases muscle building and fat burning, and therefore gives us more energy.

Regular Moderate Exercise Will Enhance Your Job Performance

Studies have proven that regular moderate exercise improves job performance. In one study, commercial real estate brokers participated in an aerobics training program for twelve weeks. They earned greater sales commissions during and after the training program than brokers who did not take part in the program.

Physically active people also process data faster. If you remain physically active, as you age you will experience a slower decline in your mental ability and speed at processing information.

Underexercising results in

Sleep disturbances	Foggy thinking
Unchecked accumulation of environmental toxins in your body	Decreased sex drive
	Decline in your mental ability to process information
Being less able to quit smoking and other addictions	Weight gain
Decreased energy and vitality	Increased anxiety, depression, and tension
Decreased decision-making abilities	Risk for atherosclerotic changes of coronary heart disease
Diminished feelings of well-being	Acceleration of the aging process
Fat gain and muscle wasting	

Regular moderate exercise results in

Deep, restful sleep	Enhanced decision-making abilities
Detoxification from environmental toxins	Enhanced feelings of well-being
Ability to quit smoking and other addictions	Fat loss and muscle building
Increased energy and vitality	Greater clarity of mind

Increased sex drive

Less decline in your mental ability to process information

More stable weight

Reduced anxiety, depression, and tension

Reversed atherosclerotic changes of coronary heart disease and unblocking of arteries

Slowing of the aging process

Regular Moderate Exercise Will Increase Your Strength, Flexibility, and Endurance

We have a vast array of exercises to choose from. No matter what exercise you choose, you will gain health benefits. If you are tired, it means that your adrenals are also fatigued. Pushing through your exhaustion with exercise will only make matters worse. If you are in a stressful period in your life, consider reducing or even avoiding vigorous exercise altogether.

Moderate Exercises

Softball, volleyball, football

Beach walking

Bowling

Cross-country skiing

Cycling

Dancing

Downhill skiing

Gardening

Golf

Hiking

Horseback riding

Ice skating

Qigong

Roller-skating or roller-blading

Tai chi

Tennis

Walking

Yoga

Strength

Unless you exercise moderately on a regular basis, you will begin to lose muscle mass after the age of thirty. After thirty, you will lose approximately three to five percent of your muscle mass every ten years. For most ambitious and highly successful people, the mental image of a weakened old body is not a reality they look forward to. Staying strong means you stay a vital, active participant in life. Optimal physical functioning and longevity are both associated with strength.

What's more, weight-bearing exercise has been proven to impede bone loss. Bone mass reaches its maximum density between the ages of twenty-five and forty. After the age of forty, bone mass declines at about one-half of a percent per year. Whatever exercise you choose, try to fit in some kind of weight-bearing activity.

Strength Training and Weight-Bearing Exercises

Aqua-aerobics	Light circuit weight training
Calisthenics such as sit-ups and push-ups	Muscle-toning fitness classes
Dancing	Walking
Gardening	Yoga

Flexibility

As we age, we lose flexibility. If your joints creak when you get out of bed in the morning, you will thank yourself in years to come for paying attention to your flexibility now. Increased range of motion, decreased risk of injury, and less creakiness and aches and pains are all associated with increased flexibility.

Yoga is probably the best activity for gaining flexibility. If you choose another exercise, it is important—both to prevent injury and to increase flexibility—to stretch before and after you exercise.

How to stretch

- Warm up for a few minutes in whatever activity you are doing

- Breathe deeply and slowly as you stretch

- Concentrate on stretching your tightest muscles

- Stretch slowly and evenly instead of bouncing. Hold stretches for thirty seconds

- Stretch again after you exercise

Endurance

It is safe to say that people who love the adrenaline rush lifestyle do not look forward to becoming old and feeble. Although a significant decline in endurance occurs after the age of forty, regular moderate exercise can prevent this decline.

Endurance exercises	
Bicycling	Long-distance walking
Hiking	Slow jogging
Kayaking	Swimming

How Long Do I Have to Exercise and How Often?

How much you need to exercise is an individual matter. Grace commented, "The worst message we have gotten over the last ten to twenty years is 'exercise at your working heart rate, for thirty to forty-five minutes three to four times a week.' In my opinion that is way too much to ask of most people and deflates their initiative to exercise before they even begin. Back in the seventies, I read that Jack La Lanne—who was the true pioneer of physical fitness in this country—said that all a person had to do was 'break a sweat' once a day. A lot of people, especially women, don't sweat very much even after an hour of vigorous exercise. His point was to exercise for ten to fifteen minutes a day. I encourage people to disregard any preconceived notions of what is optimal. You will only feel defeated. Instead, do some kind of fun exercise every day for a few minutes because it will make you feel good, make you look good, make you a happier person—and make you live longer."

Whether you are a Diehard, a Couch Potato, or anywhere in between, the goal of exercise is to come away with a sense of accomplishment and excitement and not the negativity like feeling achy, tired, angry, stupid, and fat. Exercise can clear your mind completely of worry and concerns. Often you can feel the thrill of physical activity as you engage in activities you love—gardening, beach walking, bicycling, playing with your children. Especially when recovering from adrenal burnout, it is important to exercise only to *the point of exhilaration and never to exhaustion.*

If you have been overexercising, you are the best judge of how much you can do without feeling sick, tired, and achy. If you exercise for two hours a day and you feel exhausted, cut back to one hour. Continue reducing your exercise time until you can come away from it feeling contented. If you are a Diehard and have not reached the sick, tired, and achy point yet, consider cutting back on your extreme sport. Alternate with a milder, gentler form of exercise that you can do for longer periods of time without as much stress on your adrenals.

Many people get up early in the morning to exercise, thinking that they are doing the right thing. In fact, when you are stressed or pushing the envelope too hard, vigorous exercise at any time of the day will hurt, not help you. If you are exhausted or sick, your health would benefit much more from a few extra hours of sleep.

If you are fatigued, or have been sedentary for a long period of time, any type of exercise that takes more than you already have is defeating. Very little exercise is needed to generate muscle repair. Five minutes of exercise is a good start. For example, if you choose weight training, you can begin with the tiniest amount of weight, something a little more strenuous than waving your arm. Begin with one pound or two pounds and work your way up gently. Even this small amount of stimulus will strengthen your muscles.

Exercising to exhilaration means that instead of feeling more tired you come away energized. If that means you can exercise for three minutes, then three minutes is great. If that means you can go on a fifteen-minute gentle stroll, wonderful. Allow your body the pleasure and the benefit of that recharging experience. Your body is your ultimate teacher—if you listen to it.

Normally the highest level of cortisol is in the morning, so that is naturally a great time to exercise. Cortisol levels slowly come down throughout the day just like the setting sun to allow our bodies to shift into nighttime rhythms. People who have trouble sleeping benefit most from exercising before 2 P.M.

Exercise plans for each stage of adrenal burnout

DRIVEN: One hour vigorous exercise three to five times a week.

DRAGGING: Maximum one hour vigorous exercise three times a week or one to three hours per week of rejuvenating exercise such as yoga, tai chi, dancing, or walking—not jogging.

LOSING IT: One hour rejuvenating exercise such as stretching with deep breathing, walking, yoga, or tai chi two to three hours per week.

HITTING THE WALL: Five to thirty minutes gentle rejuvenating movement such as gentle stretching or leisurely strolling one to three times per week.

BURNED OUT: Exercise is counterproductive at this stage. If you have reached Burned Out, your energy needs to be conserved. Leisurely strolling or stretching can be done for very brief periods—one to two minutes, never until you feel tired. Honor your limit now and you will begin to enjoy life again as you recover and can add more exercise.

Motivation

Your thoughts and feelings create neurotransmitters that affect your mental and physical well-being. "During the twenty years I was a jogger, I developed a habit of psyching myself up," Grace said. "Every night before I went to bed I visualized my run the following morning. When I woke up in the morning, I was ready to go out and run—no matter what. It was as if the intent was set in stone. This is still a crucial practice for me. I visualize myself hiking or doing yoga or whatever and how much I am going to enjoy it. Without fail, if I don't go through this process I face a nearly insurmountable psychological resistance."

If you think negative thoughts about yourself while you are exercising or if your thoughts are self-critical, you will create neurotransmitters that work against you. If you think *I'm too tired to exercise,* you will be too tired. If you constantly think *What's the use?* exercise probably will not do you much good. You will eventually give up and reconcile yourself to a sedentary lifestyle. Instead of letting that happen, reinforce positive beliefs about exercise. Remind yourself of how good it will make you feel and look. Tell yourself that exercise is fun. And then make it fun. Grace is an example of someone who created healthy neurotransmitters and ended up loving exercise. "Exercise has been a huge part of the enjoyment and pleasure of my life," Grace said. "I'm sure my love of exercise has both to do with the real pleasure it has brought me and probably because my years of psyching myself up have programmed me to believe that exercise is enjoyable."

Like Grace, many people do not feel comfortable working out in a gym. Exercise does not have to be in a gym. Exercise cannot be an activity that you hate. If you have tried a number of different types of exercise and feel discouraged, take heart—there are alternatives, and you will be able to find something you like to do. For example, one of my patients came to me at age sixty-one complaining of fatigue, weight gain, and lack of excitement. We talked and it was clear to me that playful exercise was missing in her life. She remembered how much she loved tap dancing as a child. After that visit she went home and took out her tap shoes—and the rest is history.

Spangler Cummings (her real stage name) found a way to make exercise fun, social, and something she looks forward to. Spangler commented, "Throughout most of my life I have taken at least one exercise class per week—yoga, ballet, modern, or tap dancing. Two years ago, a choreographer from a professional dance company asked me if I would like to join the company. At first I said that I really didn't want to perform, that I just wanted to have fun. But I decided, what the heck, life isn't a dress rehearsal. It's really been fulfilling. I am learning the dances the company knows little by little. I feel so good about myself. I feel like I am in the best shape of my life."

Spangler is an excellent example of someone who incorporated something she truly loves to do into her life—and who does not think of dancing as exercise. The thirty men and women in Spangler's dance troupe are from a mixed bag of occupations—a judge, a teacher, a statistician, a housewife, and a business manager—and range in age from their late thirties to early seventies. This is something to think about if you are feeling lonely or bored. Joining an organized group—and there are many options out there—is one way to find yourself socializing, having fun, *and* exercising on a regular basis.

Making Yourself a Priority

Some people want to exercise but cannot make themselves a priority. Chrisy Morneault, whose quest for perfection inspires her to stay up all night cleaning, explained her attitude. "I would really like to get more exercise, but if the walls need to be painted in the living room I find myself going toward the walls in the living room with a paintbrush instead of going out the door for a walk. When my husband started weight lifting and working out I thought it was unnecessary. He thinks that the hour he takes working out is something he really needs to do. I think, let's get busy and then if you are not too tired at one o'clock in the morning, you can work out."

Cleaning and work-related activities do not count as exercise. Exercise is a time for you to engage in activities that will clear your mind of concerns and give you pleasure. Like many people, Chrisy feels that work is more important than her own well-being. Short of reaching the Burned Out stage, most people do not one day awake to an epiphany that exercise is something they need to do for survival. I ask people who are resistant to making themselves a priority to take one week and dare to make their health a priority.

- Pick two or three physical activities you love such as walking, dancing, bowling, shooting baskets, playing catch, and/or gentle swimming.

- Play at any of these activities at least three times during the week for twenty to thirty minutes each time.

I am sure that after one week of moderate, regular, fun exercise you will find that you feel better afterward and have more energy. If you honestly look back at your week you will most likely have to admit that you got just as much accomplished as usual—and felt more optimistic. In fact, studies have shown that exercise increases productivity. Studies have also shown that exercise is an antidepressant and often superior to therapy and drugs.

Exercise Nutritional Tips

Contrary to recent trends in exercise advice, carbo-loading is counterproductive when trying to achieve a fat-burning metabolism. When you eat an excess of carbohydrates such as pasta, bagels, pancakes, or any refined flour–based foods, too much sugar enters your bloodstream all at once. Insulin is secreted and stores that sugar away into cells. Now that there is not enough sugar in your bloodstream, your brain assumes that you are in a time of famine and sends a red alert to your adrenals to release adrenaline and cortisol. Adrenaline releases energy from sugar stored in your liver and muscles, and cortisol *breaks down your own muscle mass* to turn it into sugar. Since excess sugar damages brain and body cells, this influx of sugar into your bloodstream triggers the secretion of insulin, which immediately stores away this new sugar away into cells. If you are in the habit of carbo-loading, day after day, your adrenals will be continually responding to red alerts from your brain, secreting adrenaline and cortisol to manage your blood sugar. Eventually your adrenal reserve will become depleted, and you can suffer from decreased muscle mass, fat around your middle, a flabby body, hypoglycemia, lowered metabolism, and premature accelerated aging.

The best diet for an athlete is a regular balanced diet of real, whole foods: protein, fat, green vegetables (an alkalinizing food), and some complex carbohydrates.

Electrolytes are minerals that are required by cells to regulate the electric charge across cell membranes. The modern diet is deficient in electrolytes, and when we exercise we sweat out even more of them. Green foods are an amazing source of natural electrolytes. I recommend that you add a green food power drink to your breakfast or as your snack on the days that you exercise to recharge your body's electrolytes. It will also give you protein and clean energy to burn like a high-octane fuel.

Power drinks, especially those made with green food, are wonderful sources of nutrients and an easy way to get protein, fiber, and essential fatty acids. (Although power drinks are mentioned throughout this book, remember that these drinks are a supplement to a balanced diet of real, whole foods—and are not meant to replace eating.) Beginning on page 334 you will find sixteen recipes for power drinks.

If after reading this you still say that you hate exercise, try to determine what it is that you really hate. Where did this dislike really come from? Often overweight people do not want anyone to see their body, and/or it feels like so much work that it is no fun. Begin by imagining ways that exercise could be fun. Often having some company helps, whether you turn on the company of TV, call up a friend, or—like Spangler—join an organized group.

When I walk, I put on a Walkman with my favorite music.

Whether it is in the gym or on the street, I get more exercise because I am having more fun listening to music. When I garden, I lift five-, ten-, and twenty-pound bags of soil. I bend over and dig for long periods of time. The lifting, digging, pulling, and sweating in a garden is great exercise for me. You do not have to engage in organized exercise, but rather do what you love to do. Anything that frees your mind and moves your body is beneficial. It could be playing vigorously with a dog for fifteen minutes or practicing your golf swing on the driving range. When you do what you love, you will gradually create a healthy habit in your life.

Exercise is only one part of your health equation. Everything you do to restore adrenal function has a cumulative effect. The more ways you try to heal yourself, the more cumulative results you will begin to enjoy. In other words, putting all your efforts into one activity, such as exercise, is not as productive as exercising a little bit and putting some of your effort into eating better, resting, and the other Simple Solutions. Instead of one big sledgehammer, a bunch of little hammers will do the job.

Simple Solution 2: Exercise Less
Tailored to your stage of burnout

Driven and Dragging

___ If you are a Diehard exerciser, consider ratcheting down your exercise program a notch or two to protect your adrenal reserves, keep your metabolism healthy, and to burn fat.

___ If you are a Diehard and love extreme sports too much to give them up, do what you can to follow all the rest of the simple solutions to protect your adrenal glands as much as possible.

___ If you are Driven by day and a Couch Potato by night (or anywhere in between), begin a moderate exercise program to protect your adrenal reserves, keep your metabolism healthy, burn fat, and keep the energy you have.

___ Incorporate strength, flexibility, and endurance exercises into your program.

___ Think positive thoughts about yourself and about exercise to create the healthy neurotransmitters that will keep you as dynamic as you are today.

___ Clear your mind of worry and concerns by doing something you love.

___ If you hate exercising in a gym, join an organized group, such as a dance troupe, to have fun.

___ Make yourself a priority when it comes to exercise—just be smart about it.

Losing It and Hitting the Wall

___ If you are a Diehard and you recognize that you are seriously Losing It or Hitting the Wall, you must exercise less even if it bruises your ego at first. Exercising less now will restore your adrenal reserves, increase your metabolism, and burn fat. In the long run, you will be back on top of your game.

___ If you are a Couch Potato or anywhere in between, a moderate exercise program will help restore your rapidly diminishing adrenal reserves, increase your metabolism, burn fat, and give you more energy.

___ Choose something fun to do that incorporates strength, flexibility, and endurance exercises.

___ Above all, be sure to exercise to exhilaration, *never to exhaustion.*

___ Think positive thoughts about yourself and about exercise to create healthy neurotransmitters.

___ Clear your mind of worry and concerns by doing something you love. If you hate exercising in a gym, join an organized group, such as a dance troupe, to have fun. Or find an exercise partner you can commiserate with. Soon you will both be having a good time and feeling much better.

___ If you do not make yourself a priority when it comes to exercise, you will soon find that you are on a slippery slope toward burnout.

Burned Out

___ Overexercising in this stage would be life-threatening. Begin to build back your strength by resting and following the other simple solutions. Have confidence that you will be back on track someday.

___ If you have been a Couch Potato, you may be able to begin exercise, very, very gently.

___ When you think positive thoughts about yourself and about exercise, you will create healthy neurotransmitters that will help you heal faster—and feel better emotionally along the way.

___ Clear your mind of worry and concerns by making meditation your exercise. Resting with your eyes closed, visualizing yourself as healed, and doing something you love will promote healthy neurotransmitters. When you do exercise, make it very gentle strolling, floating on a raft in the water, or gentle stretching.

___ Make yourself a priority when it comes to rehabilitation.

6

Simple Solution 3
Calm Your Central Nervous System

Tune down, turn on, drop out

Shortcuts to Simple Solution 3

- Learn to relax and clear your mind of concerns.

- Practice gentle yoga poses to calm
your body and mind.

- Use magnetic therapy to calm your
central nervous system.

F orty-eight-year-old Vijay Mehta speaks with an elo-
quent Indian accent, though he left his hometown
of New Delhi over twenty-five years ago. By his relaxed tone you would
not guess the hammering tempo of his life or his exhaustion. He is a
tenured university professor and international consultant and is now
also working eighteen- to twenty-hour days developing an Internet
company. "I was sitting on a plane from Los Angeles recently and the

man next to me asked me where I was going," Vijay said. "I said that I was going to stop in New York and lecture all day. I would finish the lecture at seven in the evening and then I was going to take a ten o'-clock flight to Brussels. I was going to lecture for two days in Brussels and then leave immediately and go to London and lecture for one day. Then I would come back to Los Angeles just in time to teach a class. He said, 'You know the human body is not designed to do that.' I thought that was kind of funny. And that was before I started this new Internet business. Now my schedule is even more intense."

Vijay represents hundreds and thousands of businesspeople who are now required to travel extensively to develop and maintain an international presence in our global economy. As a result of his taxing lifestyle Vijay has reached the Losing It stage. Although he avoids processed, junk, and fake foods, stimulants, and sugar and eats a diet of real, whole foods, he has neglected other areas of his health. He has stopped exercising because he does not want to make the time. He suppresses his emotions and denies himself outlets to calm his central nervous system.

"I reached a state of exhaustion where I couldn't rest and I was really wired up," Vijay explained. "At that point I was also emotionally drained. A couple of different things happened. There were times when I would try to go to sleep and I would suddenly wake up with a jerk and think that I was supposed to be giving a presentation. I would think, why am I asleep? Of course it turned out that it was one o'clock in the morning.

"I got so geared up that I actually couldn't relax or unwind. After this went on for a while, I was sitting on a plane and I felt acute pain in my chest and the pain didn't go away. I thought that I was having a heart attack. I called the flight attendant and she took my blood pressure and put me on oxygen. I was taken to an emergency room when the plane landed. When the ER doctor did all of the EKGs and things, he didn't find anything specifically wrong. He felt that it was just physical and mental exhaustion."

Vijay had experienced a panic attack. The state of sympathetic nervous system dominance uses up your calming neurotransmitters.

All that is left is an exaggerated, unbuffered surge of sympathetic neurotransmitters. Panic attacks can happen during the night and awaken you or during the day when no apparent danger is present. Shallow breathing, pounding heartbeat, feelings of impending doom, anxiety, and chest pain associated with panic attacks are caused by adrenaline. Panic attacks occur when you burn the candle at both ends and remain in a sympathetic fight-or-flight state. When you live in stress long enough, your adrenals can become overreactive and hypervigilant. There comes a point when—even if you are not in an acutely stressful situation—your adrenals will begin to pump out adrenaline. Your autonomic nervous system will not get the message to swing back to its parasympathetic state to buffer that adrenaline.

"When I went to the emergency room from the plane they had to keep all of my baggage at the airline," Vijay said. "When I got it back it had a tag with big red letters that said, *Baggage held back because passenger is in emergency room.* I kept that tag on my desk as a reminder. I thought that having it there would remind me not to work until I am exhausted."

Everyone is different. There is no scale that can be used to calculate if or when you will experience panic attacks. Some people can be in a state of sympathetic dominance for years, literally working until they drop, and never experience a panic attack. Others with the same stress level may suffer panic attacks regularly. The point is to do what you can to avoid getting into a state where panic attacks may occur.

Throughout a recent period of tragedy in my life, I had firsthand experiences of panic attacks. Mine were so acute that there were several nights when I almost called 911. I held off because, being a doctor, I knew that I was having a panic attack, not a heart attack. I decided to take my own medicine and had a direct experience with the power of 5-H GABA. You have heard the expression, "Take a chill pill." 5-H GABA and GABA are the ultimate chill pills.

5H-gamma aminobutyric acid (5-H GABA) and gamma aminobutyric acid (GABA) are amino acids that increase the amount of calming neurotransmitters in your brain. In fact, they produce the same calming effect as Valium and are used to alleviate panic attacks. The difference between 5-H GABA and GABA and Valium is that drugs such as Valium mimic our calming neurotransmitters while 5-H GABA and GABA nourish and replenish these neurotransmitters. For this reason 5-H GABA and GABA are nonaddictive. 5-H GABA is a more usable form than GABA, which is why you need a smaller dose. Both are equally effective. 5-H GABA alleviated my panic attacks in one night. I awakened the next morning almost disoriented because I was so surprised to have had such a refreshing night's sleep. On page 124, you will find formulas for preventing panic attacks.

If you are suffering from panic attacks, in addition to taking this formula, it is important to make changes in your lifestyle to improve your overall health. The first crucial step is to quit eating sugar and using caffeine, drugs, and other stimulants. Eating protein at every meal and snack will provide your body and the precursors to make serotonin, which will help you quit caffeine and other stimulants. Drinking power drinks—made with protein powder, super green food and essential fatty acids (EFAs)—is a good way to provide your body with protein and nutrients to assist in boosting serotonin. Pages 334 to 339 offer options for power drinks, and EFAs can be found on page 342.

Checklist of other actions that help raise your serotonin production and reduce the risk of panic attacks from adrenal burnout

___ Practice deep breathing, which nourishes and recharges your system while inducing relaxation and clarity. Indulge in slow, deep breathing all day long, especially before meals.

___ Provide your body with the vitamins, minerals, and other nutrients you need to repair and to loosen the stranglehold of your addiction. Your personal program can be found in chapter 9.

___ Eat balanced meals and snacks of real, whole foods to give your body the nutrients it needs to be balanced and healthy.

___ Avoid processed, junk, and fake foods and/or chemicals.

___ Do what you can to eliminate white flour and sugar from your diet.

___ Drink organic green tea, which has half the caffeine of coffee, is filled with antioxidants, and does not contain pesticides.

___ Drink detox tea.

___ Practice positive thinking to change your pyschogene.

___ Have some fun every day.

___ Engage in moderate exercise that you find fun and that clears your mind.

___ Be in sunshine every day if possible.

___ Pray and listen to inspiring music.

___ Allow your body the Three Rs: Rest, Repair, Rejuvenation.

Calming the Nervous System

In stages Driven through Burned Out, to prevent panic attacks, you can take the following formula every night before bedtime.

Panic Attack Formula

On a relatively empty stomach with something sweet such as one-quarter apple and a bite of cheese to balance the sugar, take 100 milligrams 5-H GABA. If you do not feel the calming effects after one night, increase to 200 milligrams.

or:

On a relatively empty stomach with something sweet such as one-quarter apple and a bite of cheese to balance the sugar, take 500 milligrams GABA. If you do not feel the calming effects after one night, increase to 750 milligrams.

You can find 5-H GABA and GABA at your health food store.

I recommend you begin with 5-H GABA or GABA for panic attacks. If neither alleviates your symptoms, you can add the following.

> Three times daily between meals take the following formula or one that matches as closely as possible:
> 250 milligrams kava kava
> 100 milligrams each poria sclerotium, Chinese senega root, and licorice root
>
> *or*
>
> At bedtime, take the following formula or one that matches as closely as possible:
> 150 milligrams magnesium citrate
> 75 milligrams calcium lactate
> 300 milligrams passion flower
> 150 milligrams valerian root
> 300 milligrams hops
> 150 milligrams kava kava

If these formulas do not alleviate your panic attacks, you can substitute the following (combined with either the 5-H GABA or GABA formula).

Take up to four times a day—especially at bedtime:

> On a relatively empty stomach with something sweet such as one-quarter apple and a bite of cheese to balance the sugar, take 500 milligrams L-tryptophan, by prescription only. If you do not see any improvement after two weeks, increase to maximum 1,000 milligrams.
>
> *Also add:* 25 milligrams vitamin B6.
>
> Give your body up to three weeks to experience the desired effects.

or

On a relatively empty stomach with something sweet such as one-quarter apple and a bite of cheese to balance the sugar, take 100 milligrams 5-HTP. If you do not feel the calming effects after one week, increase to 200 milligrams.

Also add: 25 milligrams vitamin B6.

Give your body up to three weeks to experience the desired effects.

You can ask your doctor for a prescription for L-tryptophan. 5-HTP can be found in any health food store.

Two other problems people have when their nervous systems are stressed out are allergies and herpes.

Allergies

Allergy formula (natural antihistamine)

Take as soon as you feel allergies coming on:

1,000 milligrams of buffered vitamin C crystals two to three times a day with 500 milligrams quercetin. If you do not see any improvement after one day, increase vitamin C to 2,000 milligrams and quercetin to 1,000 milligrams—but do not go above this. If you experience loose bowels, reduce vitamin C.

Also add: 500 milligrams B5, three times a day
and 100 milligrams nettles, one to two times a day

Vitamin C, quercetin, vitamin B5, and nettles are all available at your health food store. If this formula does not work in five days, then quit. All formulas do not work for all people.

Herpes

High cortisol levels suppress the immune system, which allows the herpes virus to come out from behind the immune barrier. In addition to the formula given here, incorporate the three Rs into your life—Rest, Repair, and Rejuvenate. Anything you can do to reduce stress will help reduce herpes outbreaks. Using magnetic therapy can prevent an outbreak and/or speed your recovery. See page 140 for more information on magnetic therapy. If herpes is causing you a lot of grief, try adding coconut to your diet. You can put coconut milk into your power drinks, make curries with coconut, and use coconut butter in place of butter. See page 82 for more on coconut oils.

> *Once a day:* 1 tablespoon coconut oil—put it in your power drink
>
> *Three times a day with meals:* 1,500 milligrams colostrum and 1,000 milligrams vitamin C and 500 milligrams lysine

Coconut products, colostrum, vitamin C, and lysine are all available at your health food store. All formulas do not work for all people. If this formula does not work in five days, then quit.

In a perfect world there would be no stress or pressure. But we are not living in a perfect world, and many enjoy pushing the envelope as they pursue their dreams. However, the human body is like any other operating system—it cannot go 24/7/365—even if you really want it

---

When you calm your central nervous system you will

Restore emotional stability

Feel safer and more
  secure

End cravings

Feel happier and better
  adjusted

Stop obsessing, worrying, and
  feeling anxious

to. Because we cannot stop the world and get off, we need to focus on easy ways to calm our central nervous systems.

Ways to Calm Your Central Nervous System

You may not be having panic attacks, but you may recognize yourself as someone who loves the adrenaline rush lifestyle. The most effective way to tame your frazzled nerves is to meditate. Since most driven people run screaming from the room at the mere mention of meditation, I like to refer to this practice as relaxation and clearing your mind. Once people feel more comfortable being in the present and with the idea of occasionally putting on the brakes in their fast-paced lives, the word *meditation* does not have such unpleasant connotations.

During the 1960s the doors to the East were flung wide open, and people in the West began to hear astonishing tales of yogis and meditation masters in India who could perform superhuman feats of bodily control and altered states of consciousness. These reports captured the attention of scientists, among them Herbert Benson, M.D., a professor at Harvard Medical School. Dr. Benson pioneered meditation in the West when he began studying yogis and meditators.

Dr. Benson discovered that meditation counteracted the fight-or-flight effect of the sympathetic nervous system. The sympathetic response to stress causes blood to be shunted to your heart, which beats harder and faster. Muscles tense, arteries constrict, and you breathe shallowly and rapidly. However, when you practice relaxing and clearing your mind, your sympathetic nervous system *tunes down* and makes it possible for the balancing act of your parasympathetic nervous system to *turn on*. Muscle tension decreases, blood pressure drops, and body temperature and metabolic rates can even drop if you prolong your practice.

As Dr. Timothy Leary used to say, "Tune in, turn on, drop out." Though he may have had a slightly different meaning, you can tune down your sympathetic nervous system, turn on your parasympathetic nervous system, and drop out of the world of your problems and concerns by practicing relaxation and clearing your mind. This practice is the most effective way to tame your central nervous system.

The practice of relaxing and clearing your mind also affects your brain waves. Commonly when you are awake and relaxed, your brain produces a pattern of smooth, regular electrical oscillations called alpha waves at a frequency of eight to thirteen cycles per second. When you are in a state of anxiety, your brain produces another waveform, called the beta rhythm, at a frequency of thirteen to thirty cycles per second. Taming your mind by focusing your thoughts will normalize your central nervous system, reduce your body's need for oxygen, and change your brain waves from the chattering beta waves to peaceful and creative alpha waves.

People who make a habit of relaxing and clearing their thoughts enjoy:

> Greater concentration/intelligence
> Creativity
> Improved ability to focus and learn
> Improved memory
> Reduced stress and anxiety
> Less incidence of disease
> Less use of alcohol and drugs
> Better cardiovascular health
> Fewer aches and pains
> Increased longevity
> More self-confidence
> Better family life
> Solid relationships
> Better job performance and satisfaction

You do not have to sit on a platform of nails, wearing a turban and chanting for an hour a day, to achieve a tranquil state. You can practice relaxing and clearing your mind anywhere or anytime during your day. *(Do not try this while driving.)* While some may choose a more traditional practice, here are four meditation techniques that you can begin with. You can practice these techniques in a quiet room of your home or your office or in your church, synagogue, or temple.

Pay Attention to Your Breath

- Sit in a chair with your feet flat on the floor, your hands resting comfortably on your thighs; or sit on the floor in a comfortable cross-legged position. You can lean against a wall for support.

- Close your eyes.

- Breathe easily in through your nose and out through your nose. Your breath will deepen naturally as your mind clears.

- Allow yourself to "watch" your breath flow in and out of your nostrils.

- If discordant thoughts creep into your consciousness, gently let those thoughts go and refocus on your breath.

Chose a Mantra/Prayer to Focus on—It Can Be the Same or Different Every Day

Here are a few suggestions:

> I am peaceful
> I am relaxed
> I am sustained by the love of God
> I am at peace with the world
> I am safe

- Sit in a chair with your feet flat on the floor, your hands resting comfortably on your thighs; or sit on the floor in a comfortable cross-legged position. You can lean against a wall for support.

- Close your eyes.

- Breathe easily in through your nose and out through your mouth, relaxing your jaw. Your breath will deepen naturally as your mind clears.

- Repeat your life-affirming thought over and over again as you practice focusing on your mantra/prayer. Any life-affirming thought that you repeat over and over again will create healthy neurotransmitters.

- If discordant thoughts creep into your consciousness, gently let those thoughts go and refocus on your life-affirming mantra/prayer.

Forward-folding relaxation

Stand with your feet hip-width apart. Take a slow, deep breath as you raise your arms overhead. When you have taken your fullest, deepest breath, begin bending at the waist. As you slowly exhale, move the crown of your head toward the floor, stretching your arms so that your palms move toward the floor. Take one long deep breath. As you are ready to inhale, slowly curl to standing, one vertebra at a time, massaging out your spine. Your head will be the last to rise; your arms will come back to your sides. Repeat. The slower you move and the deeper you breathe, the more relaxed you will become.

Relax and clear your mind through simple yoga

Another way to relax and clear your mind is by practicing gentle yoga poses. Yoga is an ancient Indian practice that unites the mind and body. Erich Schiffmann, who is the author of *Yoga: The Spirit and Practice of Moving into Stillness,* can be seen on the award-winning video "Yoga Mind & Body" with Ali MacGraw. In an interview for this book he provided the poses that follow. "There are two standing poses, one sitting twist, one sitting pose, and two poses lying down," Schiffmann said. "Notice your breathing as you practice these poses. Breathe gently, smoothly, and deeply in and out through your nose. With one movement breathe in, and with the next movement breathe out. Direct your breath to your adrenals—your lower back. Feel your lower back filling with your breath and energy. You can even repeat your mantra/prayer. These poses will leave you refreshed, exhilarated, and clear of mind.

"You might want to do these with a partner at first so that one reads the directions while the other practices the poses. When you both learn them, you can practice together. If at all possible, get up from your desk or stop what you are doing every hour or so and practice one of these poses."

During the practice of yoga, it is important to keep breathing as deeply and evenly as you can. Holding your breath, or breathing shallowly is an alarm to your body that you are in danger, signaling your body's sympathetic fight-or-flight response. So breathe deeply and allow your body to flow into the relaxing parasympathetic mode.

Simple Standing, Breathing Pose

- Stand with your legs about hip distance apart and with your feet parallel.

- Rest your hands on your waist with your thumbs placed just below your lower ribs, over each kidney.

- Take a long deep breath in and out through your nose.

- Gently rotate your thumbs in a circular motion, massaging your adrenal glands.

- Breathe deeply and imagine your cooling breath flowing into your adrenals.

- Relax and breathe deeply.

Standing Forward Fold

- Stand about a foot in front of your desk with your hands on your hips, your legs hip distance apart, with your feet parallel.

- Take a long deep breath in and out through your nose.

- Standing tall, rather than throwing your shoulders back, imagine a string attached to the crown of your head, pulling straight up so your spine elongates. Feel the trunk of your body rising away from your waist and the crown of your head reaching upward.

- On an exhale, fold gently from your hips and walk your hands across your desk.

- Cross your arms onto your desk and allow your forehead to rest on your arms.

- Feel the extension in your torso and experience your entire spine lengthening.

- Relax and listen to your breathing, deep and even in and out through your nose.

- When you are ready to rise, on an inhale, walk your hands toward you, back along the desk.

- Curl to standing, one vertebra at a time, with your head the last to rise.

If this exercise gets your heart racing, allow a few moments to rest, breathing deeply until you feel calm again, and then repeat.

Sitting Twist

- Sit sideways on an upright chair with your right hip against the back of the chair.

- Sit firmly on the entire seat with your knees and feet together.

- Imagine a string tied to the crown of your head gently pulling your torso long.

- Keep your shoulders down and back.

- On a long exhale turn right toward the back of your chair, trying not to move the position of your legs.

- Clasp the back of the chair with both hands.

- Pull with your left hand to bring your left side toward the back of the chair.

- Push with your right hand to turn your right side away from the chair.

- Keep your trunk upright, your chest moving upward, and your shoulders down.

- Gently turn your head and look over your right shoulder—only if you can do so without pain or discomfort.

- Remain calmly breathing, imagining your adrenals being flooded with cooling oxygen.

- When you are ready, release and repeat on the other side.

Child's Pose

- Kneel on the floor with your knees wide apart and your heels together.

- Lower your sitting bones to the floor if you can.

- On a long inhale, fold forward comfortably at the waist.

- Extend your arms, gently stretching your hands forward.

- Rest your forehead on the floor.

- Feel your torso moving forward away from your waist.

- Keep your sitting bones relaxing toward the floor.

- Relax and surrender into the pose and remain breathing deeply.

- When you are ready to rise, on one long inhale, curl to sitting, one vertebrae at a time, making sure that your head rises last.

Basic Sitting Pose

If your back collapses in this pose, sitting on a folded-up blanket will help. You can also sit against a wall for back support.

- Sit on the floor with your legs stretched out straight in front of you, inner knees and inner ankles touching.

- Place your palms on the floor beside your hips, fingers pointing forward.

- Straighten your elbows and gently press your palms into the floor.

- Inhale deeply and lift your rib cage, imagining a string tied to the crown of your head gently pulling upward.

- Keep your knees straight and your heels extending.

- Keep your shoulders moving back and down and your rib cage lifting.

- Open your chest and breathe deeply.

- Imagine each breath flowing into your adrenals.

- Remain until you are ready to relax.

Alternate Basic Sitting Pose with Forward Fold

You can take this pose to another level by forward folding. Forward bends help relax the nervous system by slowing your breathing and help your body move from a sympathetic to a parasympathetic state. As you rest in a forward fold, direct your breath to your adrenal glands and imagine them cooling.

- Sit in the basic sitting pose as described above.

- On a long exhalation lean forward from your hips, lift your chest, and, extending your arms, reach toward your ankles.

- Clasp your thighs, knees, shins, ankles, or feet, wherever you can easily and comfortably reach without straining.

- On an exhale, bend your elbows outward, moving the trunk of your body toward your legs and the crown of your head toward your feet.

- If you feel pain in the backs of your legs, release your stretch to where you can breathe comfortably.

- Rest in a relaxed, calm state, breathing deeply and slowly.

- When you are ready, inhale and curl to sitting.

Legs up the Wall

This pose can be done with or without blankets. If you wish to use blankets, begin by placing a pile of blankets or a bolster against the wall and sitting on it. Once you get into position, slide your body forward or back to find the position that is most comfortable for you.

- Sit on the floor, as close to a wall as possible and scoot sideways until your hip is flush with the wall.

- Swivel your buttocks toward the wall and take your legs up the wall one at a time, with your back along the floor.

- Your buttocks will be close, preferably touching the wall.

- Stretch your arms to your sides and allow them to fall outward in a relaxed position, or stretch your arms overhead.

- Relax your feet and breathe deeply.

- You may keep your legs straight up or allow your knees to bend slightly, putting the soles of your feet on the wall.

- Lie here as long as you wish to relax, breathing deeply.

- When you are ready to rise, bend your knees and turn your body to the side to slide away from the wall.

Corpse Pose

Although the corpse pose is a final relaxation pose that is done at the end of a yoga practice, it can be done any time for relaxation. In fact, this is a wonderful pose to do in bed when you find yourself unable to relax and drift into sleep. It is also a good pose in which to repeat your mantra/prayer and to practice deep, relaxing breathing.

- Lie down supine, using a pillow or folded blanket beneath your knees if you feel any lower back pain.

- You may place a pillow under your head if it feels more comfortable.

- Clasp the back of your head with your hands and pull gently, moving your chin slightly toward your chest to align your head and neck; then gently rest your head on the floor or pillow.

- Extend your legs hip distance apart and allow them to fall open naturally.

- Extend your arms at your side and allow your hands to relax.

- Draw your shoulder blades down and away from your neck so that your chest is passively open.

- Close your eyes.

- Quiet your breath, continuing to listen for its rhythmic sound.

- Remain in this pose for five to ten minutes.

- Slowly open your eyes; bend your legs and turn to your right side, using your left hand to push yourself to sitting.

Regular Naps Will Calm Your Central Nervous System

Have you ever been in a class where you were falling asleep and missed most of the information? Many people feel a slump between three and five in the afternoon. One of the signs of severely depleted adrenals is extreme mid- or late afternoon exhaustion. If you are so pooped in the afternoon that you cannot pay total attention, you make more mistakes and rob yourself of excitement and joy of life. Instead of eating sugar or drinking coffee, this is the time to eat something nutritious, nap, or exercise gently.

Napping is a powerful way to calm your central nervous system to aid in healing your adrenals. Taking a nap—even for fifteen minutes—during the midafternoon gives your adrenal glands and your biochemistry a chance to catch up. I encourage you to turn off the phone, shut the door, put your feet up on your desk, and close your eyes for fifteen minutes. Although it is not necessary to go to sleep, it certainly would be best, since napping is a short-term opportunity for your body to slide into a repair state. Breathe deeply and tell yourself, "I want to give myself this time to rest." Allow your body to relax.

If lying down is not possible, use your break time at work to go sit in a quiet place. Getting out of the office or the workplace and going for a ten-minute walk is also helpful. Getting away from aggravating stimuli is better than sitting in the midst of all of the computers, fluorescent lighting, and clatter of the workplace. If it is not possible to get away from the workplace, I encourage people to take five to twenty-five deep breaths every hour. You can set your computer or your wristwatch to remind you or put humorous stickers where you will see them to remind yourself to breathe.

Emergency Rescue for Acute Stress

Imagine you have just had the most miserable month—or two or three. Things are not going well at work. To top it off, you have family problems that are distracting and wearing you down. Heroically, you have been keeping yourself calm and together. Then one morning you awake and from the time you get out of bed, everything goes haywire.

When life just seems to be hard-balling you and you feel like a rubber band stretched to the snapping point, you do have recourse. Here are some immediate options for the short term while you are sorting out your problem.

- Have a good cry. If you are someone who bottles up your emotions, having a good cry in a moment of severe stress will allow the pressure cooker of your stress to blow off steam—even if you are a man.

- On a relatively empty stomach with something sweet, such as one-quarter apple, and a few almonds to balance the sugar, take 200 milligrams 5-H GABA—available at your health food store

    or

- With something sweet such as one-quarter apple, and a few almonds to balance the sugar, take 500 milligrams GABA—available at your health food store.

- Lie in the corpse pose—described on page 136.

- Call a therapist, priest, minister, or someone else you can talk to. Admit you need help right then and go and talk to that person immediately.

- Do something completely out of character. Take the day off from work without telling anyone what you are doing, and treat yourself. The emergency rescue lounge day activities that follow can give you some ideas.

Emergency Rescue Lounge Days Can Calm Your Central Nervous System

You might not be in the eye of the hurricane at this very moment, but we all have days when we are flat-out exhausted. You know if you try to work on these days you will spin your wheels and waste your time. I encourage you to anticipate this and create a day off once in a while. Emergency rescue lounge days are dedicated to the Three Rs: Rest, Repair, and Rejuvenation. Instead of using all of your free Saturdays or Sundays to catch up on paperwork, take one off once in a while to let your body catch up. If you have children, perhaps you can arrange for them to spend the day with relatives or friends. You can trade off with them another time to allow them an emergency rescue lounge day.

As you are running from one thing to the next, make a mental note to look forward to this day. Having good food on hand will add to your relaxation and will allow you to avoid the stress of having to go out to the store.

- Allow yourself to rest without guilt.

- Leave laundry, bill paying, cleaning, or other work for another day.

- Put your problems on hold—you cannot fix them today.

- Turn your thoughts to appreciating the good things in your life.

- Leave the newspaper for another day.

- Unplug telephones, turn off cell phones and faxes.

- Catch up with friends—avoid anyone who may bring strife into your day.

- Drink water all day.

- Reduce caffeine intake.

- Substitute for meals by eating a light snack every two hours.

- Breathe deeply and slowly as much as you can all day.

- Listen to peaceful music.

- Have a massage—preferably have the massage therapist come to your home.

- Play in your garden or go to a park, the beach, or the mountains.

- Do some gentle stretching or yoga.

- Lounge and nap.

- Watch a funny movie.

- Take a long, relaxing bath with Epsom salts or aromatherapy oils.

- Pick up a book you have had on your bookshelf but have not had time to read.

Magnetic Therapy to Calm Your Central Nervous System

Magnetic therapy is recorded in the history of many ancient civilizations. The first notation on the use of magnetism with acupuncture is found in Chinese writings circa 2000 B.C. Ancient Hindu, Egyptian, Persian, and Tibetan writings refer to the use of a lodestone—a piece of magnetite that has magnetic properties. Cleopatra is said to have worn a lodestone on her forehead to prevent aging.

For thousands of years, medical arts such as acupuncture, shiatsu (the massaging of acupuncture points), and Ayurveda (India's traditional medicine) have based their approaches on the understanding that the human body is made up of energy. Since the 1930s, researchers have recognized that the human body is influenced by the magnetic fields of the North and South Poles as well as those of the moon, sun, and other galactic fields. Scientists understood that every cell and atom of the human body is a tiny magnet, and the body has a different biochemical response to each positive and negative pole. The field of biomagnetism has since emerged, using these principles to promote healing and wellness through the energy of magnetic therapy.

Since the late nineteenth century when the industrial revolution began, scientists have recorded a decline in the strength of the earth's magnetic field. The loss is an exact ratio of oxygen loss of the planet. Think of oxygen as a lamp cord. Oxygen is what carries the earth's electromagnetic circuit. If energy were inhibited from running through the lamp cord, the light bulb in the lamp would dim. Likewise, as the earth's magnetic field diminishes, so does our metabolic functioning.

The necessity of the magnetic field to human health was realized when early astronauts and cosmonauts spent an extended period of time in space above the earth's magnetic field and suffered bone calcium loss and muscle cramps. When magnetic fields were placed in subsequent space capsules, astronauts and cosmonauts did not experience the same health problems. Just as these space travelers' metabolisms began to malfunction without the influence of the earth's magnetic field, a lowering of this field will cause a reduction in our metabolic functions and vitality. Using magnetic therapy to increase the body's electrical vitality can overcome these problems.

William H. Philpott, M.D., is a neurologist, psychiatrist, and allergist and is the author of *Magnet Therapy* (Future Medicine Publishers). He is on the Electro Magnetic Advisory Board for the National Institutes of Health. A nationally recognized authority on magnetic therapy, Dr. Philpott runs an FDA approved research program that is open to the public. In an interview for this book, Dr. Philpott said, "Humans and all living organisms are electromagnetic. The central nervous system and the peripheral nervous system function as direct current circuits with a positive magnetic field at the positive electric pole (South Pole) and a negative magnetic field at the negative electric pole (North Pole). In other words, if the compass points to the South Pole, that is the positive side to a magnet. If the compass points to the North Pole, that is the negative side to a magnet. The DNA genetic code material of each human cell has both positive and negative magnetic fields. Magnetic fields govern cell functions and are a necessary part of all physiological and psychological functions of the human body."

Dr. Peter Kulish, author of *Conquering Pain: The Art of Healing With Biomagnetism* (Fountainville Press), has a degree in advanced biomagnetics and is recognized for twenty years of research in this field. Kulish is the senior research scientist of the Magnetizer Biomagnetic Research Institute, an organization that is open to the public for health issues and wellness and for practitioner education and seminars. "The human body resembles a battery," Kulish said. "When the human battery is correctly charged up, metabolic processes function correctly. When the human battery charge is low, metabolic processes do not operate efficiently.

"The healthy body has a negative charged alkaline chemistry. Most health conditions occur over a period of time as a result of stress, bad nutrition, chemical exposure, or unhealthy electromagnetic fields. These acidic factors deplete the electricity of your body, which causes your body or a specific traumatized site on your body to become positively charged. The result is an acid state, which causes a lowering of your metabolic processes and a lowering of your immune system. Think of biomagnetism as a light switch technology. By using the proper magnetic field to switch on the energy into the body, your body chemistry can turn back to alkaline to increase your metabolism and your body's own healing abilities."

Like the earth, the human body has two polarities. The right front limbs of the body and the left back limbs of the body have a dominant positive charge. The left front limbs and the right back limbs of the body have a dominant negative charge. It is important to use negative polarity on negative zones of the body's limbs and positive polarity on positive zones of the body. "I see magnetic products in the marketplace such as mattress pads and seat cushions that have the wrong polarities," Kulish warned. "Placing magnets on your body is analogous to putting jumper cables on the battery of your car. If there is a short in your energy circuit (flow), a properly placed magnet will stimulate the correct flow of energy, helping to bring the energy circuit back to optimum health and vitality. At the same time, just as you wouldn't place battery terminals on your car backwards or it would short-circuit, the human body also has a very complicated electrochemical mechanism, which requires the same care as your car's battery. Using the wrong polarity, for example a negative magnet on a positive zone of the body, works against the normal flow of your body's electrical pathways and will create electromotive cellular chaos resulting in pain, discomfort, illness, and stress. The negative field must always go on the negative limb zone and the positive field—which is used very sparingly in specific treatments—must always go on the positive limb zone."

There are many companies selling magnetic therapy products today that do not understand the basic electromotive laws of physiology, and their products can be harmful. Magnetic therapeutic treatments are useful for specific problems and for maintaining vitality. But any constant source of the negative field, such as mattress pads, seat cushions, and shoe insoles, will cause your glands and organs to become hypoactive (underactive), which will result in the slowing down of your metabolic functioning during the time of use. Rather than constantly wearing or sleeping on magnets, think of magnetic therapy like an acupuncture treatment. Magnetic treatments are generally of short duration, and sometimes repeated throughout the day.

Below I have listed several specific treatments with the correct polarity for calming the central nervous system. If you would like to find out about further treatments for healing or pain, I have researched and trust both Philpott's and Kulish's programs and products. Both of these organizations will give you accurate guidance, which you will find on page 356. For the following treatments you will need the "Wellness Kit" from Magnetizer Biomagnetics Laboratories.

Magnetic Treatments to Calm Your Central Nervous System

Calming and energizing treatment

Repeat the following three times a day for seven to fourteen days.

- Sit in a comfortable armchair.

- At your sternum, place one "2-Stack Power Wafer" magnet negative (-) side facing your skin on the inside of your shirt and one on the outside to secure in place. Women, slip one "2-stack Power Water" negative (-) side toward your skin, inside your bra, and place one on the outside to secure in place. Your sternum is the bone indentation located at the middle of your chest.

- Place one "Super Biomagnet" on the crown of your head— above your pineal gland.

- Rest your left hand, palm side down, and your right foot on "Regular Biomagnets," negative (-) side facing your skin.

- Rest your right hand, palm side down, and your left foot on "Regular Biomagnets," positive (+) side facing your skin.

- Practice deep breathing with the magnets in place for five to ten minutes.

- After treatment, remove all magnets except the negative "2-Stack Power Wafers" over your sternum, which can be worn all day, every day until you feel fully energized. Thereafter, wear your sternum magnet three to four times a week. Remove the magnet over your sternum at night.

Insomnia treatment

- Attach "2-Stack Power Wafers" to a metal hair clip. Clip onto your hair negative (-) side facing your scalp at the crown of your head. This can raise HGH and melatonin in your brain and oxygen levels in your blood. You may use this treatment every night.

To restore adrenal function for Losing It through Burned Out

- Using plastic adhesive bandages, secure "2-Stack Power Wafers," negative (-) side facing your skin on your lower back over both left and right adrenal glands. Your adrenals are located just beneath your lowest rib on the top of your hip bones on both sides of your lower back, one to three inches on either side of your spine.

- Leave for thirty minutes, two to three times a day for four days.

For all treatments

- Drinking negative polarized water is a great way for anyone in any stage to increase energy and reduce stress. Place negative polarity magnets on your water container to energize your water. Drink at least three to four glasses a day for best results.

If you have other health problems, I recommend magnetic therapy but advise you to seek further guidance from Philpott's or Kulish's organizations, listed on page 356. Magnetic therapy should not be used by pregnant women, those with pacemakers or defibrillators, those using medical patches or insulin pumps.

Magnetic therapy, which consists of applying natural magnetic fields to the body, is beneficial and not to be confused with unhealthy electromagnetic fields that emanate from power poles, cell phones, and appliances—which is discussed on page 256.

Alkalinizing Your Body Will Calm Your Central Nervous System

Here are some habits to avoid and some to cultivate.

Acid-forming habits

Anger, rage

Complaining, nagging

Envy, obsessive jealousy

Fear and anxiety

Going without sleep

Gossip and backbiting

Hateful emotions and dreams of revenge

Lack of exercise

Overwork

Pessimism

Shallow breathing and holding your breath

Worry, fretting, and obsessing

Alkaline-forming habits

Breathing deeply

Contentment and happiness

Exercise

Fresh air

Joyful emotions and expressions of joy

Laughter

Loving and being loved

Optimism

Rest—naps, fun, play

Sleep

Yoga and other activities that help you relax and clear your mind

The techniques you have learned in this chapter will help soothe your jittery nervous system during the day, which is crucial to avoiding further adrenal exhaustion. A frazzled nervous system leads to sleep disturbances at night. Now that you understand the ways you can relax during the day, the following chapter explains the fourth Simple Solution—how you can conquer insomnia once and for all and pay off your sleep debt.

Simple Solution 3: Calm Your Central Nervous System
Tailored to your stage of burnout

Driven and Dragging

___ Since you have lots of energy and enthusiasm for learning, why not begin to develop the lifelong healthy habit of calming your central nervous system? Practice meditation to tune down your sympathetic nervous system, turn on your parasympathetic nervous system, and drop out of the world of your problems and concerns.

___ Yoga classes are cropping up everywhere. It is a practice you can easily incorporate into your day. You can do it on your own with the poses described on pages 131–137, find a class, or follow a videotape.

___ Using magnetic therapy to calm your central nervous system takes only minutes a day.

___ An occasional Emergency Rescue Lounge Days will calm your central nervous system and rest your adrenals.

___ Take a few minutes to review the acid-forming habits and alkaline-forming habits on page 146. Make the alkaline-forming habits part of your new positive thought patterns.

Losing It and Hitting the Wall

___ You know you are losing it when you start experiencing panic attacks. Instead of fretting about the shape you have gotten yourself in, take a chill pill. See page 124.

___ If you are suffering from panic attacks, follow the other simple solutions to change your lifestyle and create the healthy neurotransmitters that you need.

___ If your panic attacks are accompanied by depression and

obsessing, follow the serotonin replenishing guidelines on page 123.

___ Instead of winding up and replaying that same old mental tape of bad thoughts, doubts, and fears, you can tune down your sympathetic nervous system, turn on your parasympathetic nervous system, and drop out of the world of your problems and concerns by practicing relaxation and clearing your mind through meditation. A few minutes a day will help restore adrenal reserves.

___ You can also relax and clear your mind by practicing yoga poses. The poses described on pages 131–137 are gentle enough for even the most uptight body. You will soon be feeling so good you will be looking around for a class to join.

___ Let's not mess around with your health at this point. You can calm your central nervous system and aid in healing your adrenals by taking naps or break times during the day—and avoid hitting the wall.

___ Practice occasional Emergency Rescue Lounge Days to calm your central nervous system and rest your adrenals. You will love every minute of it.

___ Use magnetic therapy to calm your central nervous system.

___ Acid-forming habits are a sure way to plunge you deeper into burnout. Review the alkaline-forming habits found on page 146 and begin practicing positive behaviors.

Burned Out

___ If panic attacks have become part and parcel of your life, avoid the next one by taking a chill pill—see page 124.

___ Review this chapter again and give it some thought while you are resting and thinking about ways to take care of your-SELF.

___ You cannot reach burnout and still have a good supply of serotonin. You can begin to replenishing your brain's serotonin reserves by following the formula found on page 123.

___ Now is a crucial time to practice meditation. Tune down your sympathetic nervous system, turn on your parasympathetic nervous system, and drop out of the world of your problems and concerns by practicing relaxation and clearing your mind.

___ Even the most burned out can practice some of the gentle yoga poses described on pages 131–137. These poses will make you feel much more hopeful.

___ There is nothing stopping you from calming your central nervous system and aiding in healing your adrenals by taking regular naps or break times every day. Two naps would not be considered indulgent. Go ahead and take care of yourself.

___ Now you can indulge in regular Emergency Rescue Lounge Days to calm your central nervous system and rest your adrenals.

___ Use magnetic therapy regularly to calm your central nervous system.

___ Acid-forming habits are part of your past now. From this day forward, make your best effort to practice alkalinizing habits.

Simple Solution 4
Pay Off Your
Sleep Debt

*Mom was right when she said
that things would look
better in the morning*

Shortcuts to Simple Solution 4

- Make sleep a priority and cultivate healthy sleep habits.

- Stop eating sugar at night.

- Take sleep supplements, if needed.

In 1974, twenty-eight-year-old Madeline Sparrow and her husband answered a tiny ad in the classifieds offering land "on the rim of the world." The couple and their four young children subsequently moved into a one-room cabin on thirty-five acres sprawled across a mountain ridge. Madeline, now a fifty-five-year-old drama teacher, sat on a couch in front of a picture window that framed the breathtaking view of the Pacific Ocean she has enjoyed for twenty-six years.

Slender and attractive with a flair for the artistic, Madeline is an intense actress who speaks in *italics*. "People called us hippies, but we *hated* that name," Madeline said. "We weren't doing drugs or anything like that. We were living an alternative lifestyle. We grew a huge vegetable garden and had a cow that we milked, so we had milk and cream and cheese. My greatest time was when the kids were real young. I stayed home with them and we put on plays at school. We were all natural, playing with the kids outdoors. I had sleep problems then, but since I've gotten older, it's gotten worse. The slightest little sound wakes me up and I'm wide-awake, and my mind starts racing. I lie there in the dark with nothing but my thoughts. I just toss and turn for hours and finally get to sleep in the morning when it's time to get up. For the last twenty years I've gotten about four hours of interrupted sleep a night."

Madeline has been spared the noise, pollution, and stress of city life for over a quarter of a century. Living in the country on a farm, she has eaten mostly natural foods. She has religiously taken a forty-five-minute mountain walk six days a week. In these and other ways, she has lived a healthy life. Madeline, who is now in the Hitting the Wall stage, is a case of someone entering the burnout stages later in life. The stress of her career began in the past fifteen years as her children left home and she went to work in the theater. "Theater is not bad stress, but it's very intense," Madeline said. "I teach *pubescent teenagers*. Working with kids all the time is one of my greatest loves and one of my greatest hates. When it's good it's good and when it's hard it's *hard*." Madeline has her hands full in a craft that is intense and taxing. Added to this, her body has been stressed to near burnout because of her insomnia. She attributes her lifelong insomnia to the fact that she is a "worrywart." She is suffering now from undiagnosable maladies, such as intestinal problems, intermittent fevers, and debilitating muscle cramps, that are thought to have roots in an autoimmune condition. It is likely that her health problems stem from years of sleep deprivation.

Millions of people like Madeline would love to get to sleep, but they suffer from insomnia—the inability to fall asleep or to remain asleep restfully through the night or awakening too early. Sleep is as crucial to survival as eating and breathing. Find out how you stack up in your sleeping patterns.

Are you sleep deprived?

Check all that are true.

___ You have nightmares.

___ You need an alarm clock to awaken you—and you put it across the room.

___ You hit the snooze button two or three times.

___ You awaken tired and drag yourself out of bed.

___ It takes two to four cups of coffee to get you going in the morning.

___ You have a hard time concentrating and remembering things during the day.

___ You eat sugar for energy.

___ You are often irritable and cranky.

___ You have a hard time focusing on tasks, problem-solving, and being creative.

___ You fantasize about sleeping and look forward to a good night's sleep.

___ You often fall asleep watching TV.

___ You often fall asleep after heavy meals or after little alcohol.

___ You often fall asleep easily after dinner but cannot fall asleep later in bed.

___ You often feel drowsy while driving.

___ You often sleep extra hours on weekend mornings.

___ You have dark circles under your eyes.

If you checked two or more of these factors, you are probably showing signs of a sleep problem. Carrying a substantial sleep debt has contributed to the epidemic of adrenal burnout in this country. Insomniacs often develop insomnia as a result of their psychogene, or learned beliefs and fears. Madeline, whose "whole family has some sort of sleep disorder," described her psychogenic conditioning. "My mother was a German Lutheran who was as pure as the driven snow. She was always taking care of other people and making sure they were happy. Her house was perfect. If you looked in her dresser drawers, they were perfect too. I grew up listening to nice music like Lawrence Welk and watching nice TV shows like *Leave It to Beaver* and *Donna Reed* and hearing my parents constantly tell me that I was a bad and selfish girl and that I should be good."

Madeline's psychogenic belief was that she had to be good to be loved, and her fear that she was not good enough → led to worry and feeling apologetic about her perceived failings → led to trying to please everyone at the expense of sabotaging her artistic accomplishments → led to insomnia and autoimmune conditions.

If you suffer from insomnia, it might be useful here for you to examine your psychogene equation and try to determine what is keeping you awake at night.

What is your psychogene equation?

_____→ led to

What is your psychogene—your beliefs and fears?

_____→ led to

What emotion can you identify with your psychogene?

_____→ led to

What behaviors have you developed in an attempt to appease that emotion?

_____

What emotional or physical symptoms have you developed as a result? Is insomnia part of your equation?

The study of psychoneuroimmunology (PNI) (*sigh ko nur-o im you nol agee*), has helped us understand that our thoughts and beliefs can influence our sleep. Your body's biochemistry is heavily influenced by what you think, feel, and believe. It is not so black and white that we can say that a certain belief or fear produces a specific kind of neurotransmitter, which leads to insomnia. But we do know that if we think enough negative thoughts about sleep, we will create neurotransmitters that will result in insomnia. The twenty years Madeline has spent thinking and verbalizing thoughts such as *Well, here goes another sleepless night* or *I'm a hopeless insomniac* have created unhealthy neurotransmitters, which are now dictating sleeplessness. It is a double whammy. She has her psychogene beliefs and fears that contribute to her insomnia, and she has the neurotransmitters that exacerbate those beliefs and fears.

On the other hand, if Madeline were to think *I am going to sleep*, she would eventually produce healthy neurotransmitters, which would aid in making her drowsy and sleepy.

Nighttime sleep is the natural time for your body to slip into the biochemistry of repair. While you sleep your body is Resting, Repairing, and Rejuvenating—rebuilding its reserve so that you wake up with more of it than you went to sleep with. Your mother was right when she said that things would look better in the morning. Everyone knows how much better they feel physically and mentally after a deep sleep. You are better equipped to take on the day when you have had a good night's rest. In fact, paying off your sleep debt is

Some of the Benefits of Becoming Healthier

Sleeping deeply and restfully every night

Ending insomnia

Instead of dragging around exhausted, having energy to burn

Your nightmares will stop and you will have pleasant dreams

You will no longer need to trek to the bathroom all night long one important step to avoiding burnout. The healthier you get, the better your sleep will become. Following Simple Solutions 1, 2, and 3—eating whole foods, exercising appropriately, and calming the central nervous system—will start you on the way to being able to achieve Simple Solution 4: paying off your sleep debt to repair tired adrenals.

People are aging quickly today because they do not give their bodies, and especially their adrenal glands, an opportunity to repair. Think of your body's reserves as a bank account. Your adrenal glands have only so much reserve. Eventually, if you continue to spend that reserve, without allowing interest to accrue, your adrenals will not be able to keep up with the demand and your account will run dry. You cannot go go go go go and then sleep in on one morning a week and expect to restore your depleted reserves. Your body and your adrenals need nightly doses of the Three Rs: Rest, Repair, and Rejuvenation. Just as you cannot fix a flat tire while you are riding your bicycle, your adrenal glands cannot Rest, Repair, and Rejuvenate when they are constantly responding to demand. Taking the time and making the effort to change your sleep habits will improve your overall health and the quality of your life and give you the self-confidence and energy to be successful in all your pursuits.

Adequate sleep reduces the risk of heart attack, immune disorders, diabetes, depression, and fatigue. It is natural for the body to sleep and repair. It is not natural not to sleep. So you have your body's natural operating system on your side. To end your insomnia, you have to want to do things differently, and you must believe that you can do it. Your positive attitude will influence your body to create the neurotransmitters that will aid in sleep. When you think positive thoughts about sleep, your body will get better at creating what I call the biochemistry of sleep. The following solutions can help you create a biochemistry of sleep and end your insomnia.

Living in a Sympathetic (Daytime)-Dominant State:

People who love the sensation of the adrenaline rush live in a heightened state of sympathetic nervous system adrenal excess. To your body, living in a sympathetic-dominant state is like being continually chased by a tiger in the woods.

Behaviors that result in a state of sympathetic dominance and contribute to insomnia

Skipping meals/dieting

Eating processed, junk, or fake foods

Not exercising or exercising too much

Avoiding or neglecting relaxation and other ways to calm your central nervous system

Blowing past your own fatigue to finish the day's work

Not getting enough sleep

Using sugar, caffeine, nicotine, drugs, or herbal stimulants to function at a higher rate when you are already tired

Breathing shallowly when tense, instead of breathing deeply

Exposing yourself to toxins in the environment, household products, and food

Worrying

Mentally replaying stressful inner dialogues

Neglecting fun and relaxing activities that allow you to clear your mind

Putting yourself last

In this day and age, it may be difficult to emerge completely from sympathetic dominance. Fears of never being enough, never doing enough, never having enough, anxiety over being late for an appointment, of overspending on our credit cards, of having a fight with our spouse or boss, and on and on all contribute to the sympathetic-dominant state. Skipping a meal is perceived as a dangerous time of famine by your body, and your adrenals will pump out stress hormones in an attempt to help keep you alive. We are surrounded by cataclysmic noises from television, the backfiring of engines, and the blare of traffic, sirens, and car alarms, which signal our adrenals that we are in imminent danger. The workplace has changed, and many people today use air travel the way people in the year 1900 used streetcars. All of these stress factors add up.

Sleep is the natural time for the systems of your body to Rest, Repair, and Rejuvenate, to allow the alkaline tide to balance the acidity your body accumulated during the day. Living in a state of sympathetic dominance prevents the natural ebb and flow of the pendulum of the autonomic nervous system and the alkaline tide at night. Incorporating as many of the Ten Simple Solutions into your life as possible will help your body's autonomic nervous system to easily adjust from a sympathetic to a parasympathetic state. It will aid in ending your insomnia.

What it will feel like when you start getting regular deep sleep

You will awaken in the morning refreshed and ready to take on the day.

You will feel calmer and more in control.

Your mind will be clear, and your thoughts will be sharp.

Your sex drive will return.

You will be able to problem-solve.

You will feel creative again.

You will feel alert while driving.

You will not need those extra sleeping-in hours on the weekend.

You will be in a good mood and will feel generous toward yourself and others.

Sleep Recommendations

In each progressive stage of adrenal burnout, your need for rest and sleep increases. Recommendations for each stage follow. You may not believe the amount of sleep and rest you need now because you have always gotten along on so much less. Or maybe you have suffered from insomnia for so long that you doubt that you can sleep. As you begin to make small changes using the Ten Simple Solutions, you will be more able to get a good night's rest. Resting during the day is also a key factor in restoring adrenal function. Remember, you are legally entitled to two coffee breaks. Instead of coffee, I suggest retreat periods. A Japanese study showed that if workers took their two fifteen-minute breaks a day, they were more productive than if they had worked straight through.

Driven

NIGHTTIME: Six to eight hours

DAYTIME: Nap as needed—go ahead and indulge yourself—you are worth it.

Dragging

NIGHTTIME: Eight hours

DAYTIME: Ten to fifteen minutes of quiet retreat, such as going for a walk or closing your eyes for ten minutes. Go into the restroom, close the door, and rest or meditate there if you cannot find another private place. If you are at home, no TV, peaceful music only.

Losing It

NIGHTTIME: Eight hours is critical at this stage.

DAYTIME: Two ten- to fifteen-minute quiet retreat periods is the minimum, such as going for a walk or closing your eyes for ten minutes. Go into the restroom, close the door, and rest or meditate there if you cannot find another private place. If you are at home, no TV, peaceful music only.

Hitting the Wall

NIGHTTIME: Eight to nine hours is critical now.

DAYTIME: Two ten- to fifteen-minute quiet retreat periods is the minimum, such as going for a walk or closing your eyes for ten minutes.

Go into the restroom, close the door, and rest or meditate there if you cannot find another private place. If you are at home, no television, peaceful music only.

Burned Out

At this stage, your health is in a delicate balance, so if at all possible, take a leave of absence, go on disability, or at most, work part-time.

NIGHTTIME: Eight to ten hours is critical.

DAYTIME: Fifteen to thirty minutes restful retreat three times a day, napping in a serene environment. If you are at home, try to avoid TV entirely. Instead listen to peaceful music and meditate.

Poor Sleep Habits

It may be that you have simply cultivated insomnia by indulging in bad habits. With a little effort you can turn your problem around.

During the day your brain retains everything you see and experience. At night, your brain repairs itself, makes new connections, and creates order out of the information you have taken in during the previous day. Research suggests that rapid eye movement (REM) sleep, which is associated with dreaming, is the time the brain integrates information taken in during the day and consolidates new knowledge into long-term memory. It is very much like when our computer is taking information from RAM and consolidating it onto our hard drive. According to sleep expert James Maas, M.D., "Between the seventh and eighth hour is when we get almost an hour of rapid eye movement (REM) sleep, the time when the mind repairs itself, grows new connections, and puts it all together. REM sleep occurs about every ninety minutes, and the periods of REM sleep get longer as the night progresses. If you're a six-hour sleeper, you're missing that last, important opportunity to repair and to prepare for the coming day."

When you do not sleep enough, or when your sleep is sketchy, you shortchange your brain's opportunity for creative processing.

When you do not sleep enough, your brain carries a backlog of information. When you finally do get to sleep, your brain will launch dreams in an attempt to process this stored information. Disruptive dreams may constantly awaken you. "I usually sleep for a couple of hours, then I wake up like someone jolted me out of bed," Madeline commented. "I'll be wide-awake. My heart pounds, and I'm just *awake awake awake*. I've been desperate, but I decided not to use sleeping pills even though I have been tempted at times." Madeline was wise. Sleep medications suppress REM sleep. Often the longer someone takes sleep medication the harder it will be for that person to get to sleep because there is so much backlogged information waiting to be processed—or the information will awaken the person and/or make the sleep more restless.

The pineal gland is a pea-sized organ housed deep in the brain that identifies day and night by sensing light and dark. It regulates the body's circadian rhythm, a daily rhythmic activity cycle, based on twenty-four-hour intervals. The pineal gland produces the hormone melatonin in periods of darkness, which makes you feel sleepy and aids in turning on the nighttime repair and rejuvenation processes. Sleep experts recommend that people go to bed as soon as possible after sundown because this is the time that your pineal gland registers dark and your brain will receive a sleep-inducing infusion of melatonin. Melatonin is suppressed when you are in light. If you are up late at night under artificial lights—even the light from the TV— the release of melatonin will be inhibited. Electricity has encouraged most people to stay up far beyond the time when their bodies would prefer to go to sleep.

Another hormone that is released primarily at night by your pituitary gland is human growth hormone (hGH), which acts as the conductor to orchestrate the processes of repair and helps rebuild lean body mass—muscles and bone. When your body does not regularly produce hGH, your body does not repair as well or as fast, which results in premature aging.

At night our autonomic nervous system is supposed to move from the acidic, sympathetic state of breaking down to the alkaline, parasympathetic state of building up. Our ancestors sat by the light of a fire, which allowed their internal rhythm to slow down before they drifted off to sleep. Most of us do not go to sleep within two hours of sunset. Instead we stay up watching TV, working, arguing, surfing the Internet, drinking caffeine, paying bills, doing the laundry, eating sugar, and so on. Too often we go to bed wound up, unable to drift into quality sleep; and so we remain in a heightened state of sympathetic dominance, which leads to adrenal exhaustion.

Depriving your body of sleep prevents the return of the alkaline tide and ultimately contributes to panic biochemistry. The state of sympathetic dominance is made more extreme by lack of sleep. During sleep our calming neurotransmitters are regenerated. Insomnia causes a deficit of calming neurotransmitters. Chronic insomnia compounds this deficit until we do not have enough calming neurotransmitters to put us to sleep, to keep us asleep, or to buffer the challenges of the day.

Activities to Avoid After Dinner

Answering emails

Arguing

Cleaning

Drinking caffeine

Eating sugar

Exercise

Figuring out your budget/taxes

Laundry

Leftover tasks from the day or from work

Paying bills

Puttering in your garage

Reading upsetting or scary books

Staying awake past drowsiness to play video/computer games

Staying awake past drowsiness to watch TV or movies

Surfing the net

Talking on the phone

Working on a project such as painting or sewing

Writing letters—especially if they are agitating

After-dinner activities that will promote sleep

Having pleasant
   conversation
Going for a gentle stroll
Reading a good book

Listening to relaxing music
   and/or positive imagery
   tapes
Meditating

If you have developed poor sleep patterns, now is a good time to start improving your sleep habits. It is possible to cure this type of insomnia, but it may take some practice. If you have spent ten, twenty, or thirty years staying up to watch the late show on TV, it will take some time to learn new habits. The first step in curing your insomnia is to believe that you can. The next step is to begin to change your habits. Why not make it a priority? Your total health will be improved with sleep.

Watching television before bed keeps your brain surprisingly stimulated, given the insipid quality of nighttime TV programming. When you use your bedroom for activities other than sleep, such as reading, eating, talking on the phone, or watching TV in bed, you begin to unconsciously associate your bedroom with wakefulness.

Make your bedroom your sanctuary

Use your bedroom only for sleep and lovemaking
Avoid bill paying, eating, or reading in bed
Remove your telephone and/or TV from your bedroom

Nighttime Obsessing

"I would say that most of my sleep problems are due to the fact that I'm a worrywart," Madeline admitted. "I just mull over things when I wake up in the middle of the night. My insomnia used to be caused by something specific that was causing me anxiety. Now everything seems to cause me anxiety, including someone else's problems. I've allowed this worrying to become a habit that just feeds on itself." Not being able to fall asleep because of obsessive thoughts or awakening to obsess is a common factor in people not getting adequate sleep.

Inability to fall asleep or awakening in the night is often caused by adrenal hysteria—when the adrenals turn on at the wrong time. When you remain in a sympathetic-dominant state, your autonomic nervous system cannot flow into the restful repair of the parasympathetic state. The communications network between your pituitary and your adrenals is disrupted. Your adrenals are not being suppressed at night as they should be but instead are activated to secrete adrenaline, cortisol and DHEA. These high levels of adreneline, cortisol and DHEA are appropriate during the day but are stimulating at night.

Phosphatidylserine, which is a brain nutrient, helps rebalance pituitary/adrenal communication and nourishes and supports your adrenals while you rest. For those who suffer from insomnia because their adrenals are turning on inappropriately at night, phosphatidylserine can help. You know this is happening when you routinely awake in the middle of the night once, twice, or more times a night. You may experience your heart beating rapidly and/or you have to get up and go to the bathroom all night long. Phosphatidylserine influences your brain's messages to your adrenals so that they stop the inappropriate release of adrenaline, cortisol, and DHEA.

If your thoughts are so powerful that you find that you are feeling restless—an adrenaline response—you do have recourse. Begin by taking 100 milligrams of phosphatidylserine at bedtime. If you do not see any improvement within two days, increase to 200 milligrams phosphatidylserine. You can find phosphatidylserine at your health food store.

There are a few time-honored ways to relax the body so that you can rest. Yoga is full of answers. One suggestion is to try the corpse pose.

Corpse pose and combined breathing
to get back to sleep

- Lie on your back, with a pillow or folded blanket beneath your knees if you feel any lower back pain.

- Clasp the back of your head with your hands and pull gently, moving your chin slightly toward your chest, to align your head and neck; then gently rest your head on your pillow.

- Extend your legs hip distance apart and allow them to fall open naturally.

- Extend your arms at your sides and allow your hands to relax.

- Draw your shoulder blades down and away from your neck so that your chest is passively open.

- Close your eyes.

- Breath as deeply and evenly as you can. Holding your breath, or breathing shallowly is an alarm to your body that you are in danger, signaling your body's sympathetic fight-or-flight response. So breathe deeply and allow your body to flow into the relaxing parasympathetic mode.

- Repeat a positive thought like a prayer. Say to yourself, "Everything is going to be all right."

Calming yourself by practicing the corpse pose while breathing and repeating a mantra/prayer helps to create a peaceful, healing biochemistry. Thinking positive thoughts while breathing deeply and slowly is a conscious way of telling your brain what you want it to do—and it can lull you to sleep. Since every thought influences the production of neurotransmitters, positive thoughts have a cumulative positive influence. Over time you will experience less agitation at night.

When you awake in the morning, it is important for you to

recognize and consciously give yourself credit and affirm that what you did made a difference. Say to yourself, "I did it. I fell asleep."

Muscle Spasms

Madeline's long history of sleep deprivation has led to various autoimmune conditions that have defied diagnosis and treatment. Studies have shown that chronic sleep loss accelerates aging and increases the severity of age-related ailments such as diabetes, hypertension, obesity, and memory loss. Madeline suffers from muscle spasms that appear to have roots in her autoimmune disorder. "My legs and arms ache all the time, and I have these weird spasms in my feet and legs and in my hands, and now I'm getting them once in a while under my rib cage."

If you are kept awake by muscle spasms, it is often due to a mineral deficiency. Potassium, magnesium, and calcium are the most commonly missing minerals, especially in older people who are malnourished from years of eating processed, junk, and fake foods. Magnesium is the most well-known muscle relaxant. In fact, some heart attacks include spasms in the coronary arteries and can be stopped by administering intravenous magnesium. Magnesium is such a powerful muscle relaxant that it is used in labor and delivery to stop premature labor. In my practice I use intravenous magnesium to rid people of their asthma attacks, which are lung muscle spasms; heart palpitations, which are blood vessel and muscle spasms; and pelvic pain and menstrual pain, which are pelvic muscle spasms.

Sixty to seventy-five percent of Americans are magnesium deficient. Magnesium supplements can help calm your muscle spasms and make you a healthier, calmer person. You will have an easier time getting to sleep and staying asleep.

Thirty minutes before bedtime, take 100 to 200 milligrams of magnesium glycinate—reduce the dose if you experience loose bowels. You can find magnesium glycinate at your health food store.

Eating Sugar at Night

Eating sugar at night, including drinking alcohol, which is all sugar, interferes with your body's circadian rhythm by stimulating your adrenal glands at the wrong time. After eating sugar, your pancreas releases a surge of insulin, which causes your blood sugar to drop precipitously. This drop sends a red alert from your brain to your adrenals to release adrenaline in an attempt to rescue your sinking blood sugar. Instead of Resting, Repairing, and Rejuvenating in preparation for the next day, your adrenals are pumping out stress hormones, which will keep you awake and may even cause night sweats and nightmares.

Eating sugar at night has all the backlash ramifications of eating sugar during the day, with the added negatives of insomnia and the suppression of the release of hGH by your pituitary gland. HGH helps balance all the other systems in the body and is the most potent longevity hormone known. HGH accelerates repair and stimulates muscle building and fat burning. Because muscle mass dictates the rate of metabolism, when you have more muscle mass, you have more energy. The more sugar you eat at night, the harder it is for your body to rejuvenate and repair and the more likely you are to put on weight around your middle. Ironically, when your body produces hGH at night, it stimulates fat burning. Your midsection fat is the fat it is most likely to burn. I joke with my patients that if you eat a lot of sugar at night, you might as well just apply it to your hips because you cannot burn it while you sleep.

You can try the "Grandmother Method" to help this problem: Switch to a bedtime snack of protein, especially turkey, cottage cheese, or organic, raw milk, which will provide your body with tryptophan. Tryptophan is the precursor to melatonin, the hormone that aids in sleep, and to the amino acid tyrosine, which is a mood elevator. When we eat the right bedtime snack, our bodies can more readily alter our brain biochemistry to put us to sleep.

Prescriptions for Sleep

Our brain's ability to make the hormone melatonin decreases with age, as in the case of so many other hormones. If you are suffering from insomnia, taking melatonin is a good next step. Begin by taking one milligram of melatonin at bedtime. If one milligram does not make you sleepy and help keep you asleep all night, increase by one milligram per week as needed, up to five milligrams. While melatonin has been tested and found to be extremely safe, there are those who have a paradoxical reaction wherein melatonin causes them to feel energized or to have nightmares. This is not life threatening, but it is obviously not the goal, so also try the other formulas recommended here. You can find melatonin at your health food store.

Therapeutic amounts of amino acids can replenish your neurotransmitters to aid in sleep and also help alkalinize your body.

If you have been on a strict no-salt diet, simply adding up to one quarter teaspoon of sea salt to your daily diet may help with insomnia. *This advice is not meant to contradict the advice of your doctor.*

When You Cannot Sleep Because of Obsessive Thoughts

Your insomnia may be caused by obsessive thoughts that keep you restless and wide awake. Two categories of insomnia formulas follow to help calm you and put you to sleep. One is for immediate relief, and the other is to correct insomnia in the long term. It may take up to one month for you to notice the effects of the long-term formula. You may begin a short-term formula and a long-term formula at the same time. As your sleep improves, omit the short-term formula.

Short-term Relief from Insomnia and Nighttime Waking with Obsessive Thoughts

5-H gamma aminobutyric acid (5-H GABA) and gamma aminobutyric acid (GABA) are amino acids that increase the amount of calming neurotransmitters in your brain. You have heard the expression

"Take a chill pill." 5-H GABA and GABA are the ultimate chill pills. In fact, they produce the same calming effect as Valium and are often used to alleviate panic attacks. The difference between 5-H GABA, GABA, and Valium is that drugs such as Valium mimic our calming neurotransmitters while 5-H GABA and GABA nourish and replenish these neurotransmitters. For this reason 5-H GABA and GABA are nonaddictive. 5-H GABA is a more usable form than GABA, which is why you need a smaller dose.

Thirty minutes before bedtime:

On a relatively empty stomach with something sweet such as one-quarter apple and a bite of cheese to balance the sugar, take 100 milligrams 5-H GABA. If you do not see any improvement within two weeks, increase to 200 milligrams.

or

On a relatively empty stomach with something sweet such as one-quarter apple and a bite of cheese to balance the sugar, take 500 milligrams GABA. If you do not see any improvement after two weeks, increase to 1,000 milligrams.

You can find GABA or 5-H GABA at your health food store.

If GABA or 5-H GABA do not put you to sleep, you can switch to:

Phosphatidylserine—100 milligrams. If you do not see any improvement after two nights, increase to 200 milligrams phosphatidylserine.

If phosphatidylserine does not work alone, you can also add the following formula or one that matches as closely as possible:

300 milligrams passion flower
150 milligrams valerian root
300 milligrams hops
150 milligrams kava kava root

or

1 milligram melatonin—within three hours after dark. If you do not see any improvement after one week, increase to 2 milligrams for another two weeks, up to 5 milligrams.

Long-term Relief from Insomnia and Nighttime Waking with Obsessive Thoughts

Take 30 minutes before bedtime:

Phosphatidylserine—100 milligrams. If you do not see any improvement after two days, increase to 200 milligrams phosphatidylserine.

If phosphatidylserine does not work alone, you can also add one of the following formulas:

1 milligram melatonin—within three hours after dark. If you do not see any improvement after one week, increase to 2 milligrams for another week, up to 5 milligrams.

or

Take the following formula or one that matches as closely as possible:
300 milligrams passion flower
150 milligrams valerian root

or

On a relatively empty stomach, with something sweet such as one-quarter apple and a bite of cheese to balance the sugar, take 100 milligrams 5-H GABA. If you do not see any improvement after two weeks, increase to 200 milligrams.

or

On a relatively empty stomach, with something sweet such as one-quarter apple and a bite of cheese to balance the sugar, take 500 milligrams GABA. If you do not see any improvement after two weeks, increase to 1,000 milligrams.

or

On a relatively empty stomach, with something sweet such as one-quarter apple and a cup of warm raw milk to balance the sugar—500 milligrams of L-tryptophan—by prescription only. If you do not see any improvement within two weeks, increase to 1,000 milligrams.

Also add: 25 milligrams vitamin B6.

or

On a relatively empty stomach, with something sweet such as one-quarter apple and a cup of warm raw milk to balance the sugar, take 100 milligrams 5-HTP. If you do not see any improvement after two weeks, increase to 200 milligrams.

Also add: 25 milligrams vitamin B6.

or

Two sprays orally of homeopathic human growth hormone.

Human Growth Hormone (hGH) helps balance all the other systems in our body and is the most potent longevity hormone known. The natural decline of human growth hormone often parallels aging and burnout. The replacement of hGH secretion has been observed to regenerate and repair most systems including adrenals.

You may take these formulas to your health food store and research the products that match them as closely as possible. Homeopathic human growth hormone can be obtained through your health care practitioner. You can ask your doctor for a prescription for L-tryptophan. 5-HTP, 5-H GABA, GABA, and melatonin are all available in health food stores.

Checklist to change your sleep
biochemistry and be great in bed

___ Eat dinner at least two hours before bedtime.

___ Go to bed as long before midnight as possible.

___ Avoid alcohol before bedtime. Alcohol has a boomerang effect. It can lull you to sleep, but when your blood sugar crashes, you will awaken with a start and may not be able to fall back asleep.

___ Have a cup of Sleepytime tea, which contains the soothing, calming, relaxing herbs chamomile, spearmint, and lemongrass along with tilia flowers, blackberry leaf, hawthorn berries, and rosebuds.

___ Go to bed when you are initially tired and feel sleepy.

___ Listen to relaxing music

___ Take a bath with one or two cups Epsom salts, which is hydrated magnesium sulfate—available in any drugstore. This will allow your body to calm as the magnesium is absorbed through your skin. Warming your core body temperature will make you drowsy.

___ Keep your bedroom temperature at 68 degrees, which corresponds with your lowest body temperature during sleep.

___ Darken your bedroom as much as possible or wear eye shades—available at any drugstore.

___ If your mattress is lumpy or uncomfortable, invest in a new mattress.

___ Try to get up at the same time every day—within one hour.

Caffeine

If consuming caffeine is causing your insomnia—whether from drinking coffee, tea, or sodas—wanting to feel better is a big part of breaking this addiction. People use this drug to wake up in the morning, to keep going all day, and to give them a boost when they begin to drag. But if you have insomnia and suffer from fatigue, you already know that your drug is not working. It is time to try another approach.

If you quit caffeine abruptly, you may feel weak, headachy, fatigued, and nauseated and have cravings. Please back off coffee gently, use the serotonin-boosting formula that follows, and take the supplements recommended in chapter 9 for your stage of burnout. Not only is the demand gradually decreased but your craving will gradually diminish, and your adrenals will repair and begin to respond again. Weaning yourself slowly off coffee will allow you to feel better along the way instead of suffering from withdrawal symptoms. Begin by giving up one-half cup of coffee every few days. If you drink three cups of coffee a day, then you can quit in two to three weeks. If you drink ten cups, it may take you up to two months to quit entirely. To help keep from slipping back into old habits, before you begin mark your calendar each week as a reminder of how many cups of coffee you will drink each day that week.

Switching to decaffeinated coffee is not the same as quitting, since decaffeinated coffee still contains caffeine. In addition, except for Swiss water-processed decaffeinated coffee, most coffees are decaffeinated with methylene chloride, a carcinogen, which you then ingest with your decreased caffeine.

I also encourage you to ask less of yourself during this healing time. Realize that there is a repair process going on. Quitting an addiction like caffeine is a process in which you must be gentle with yourself.

Checklist for other factors that will help raise your serotonin production

____ Eat protein at every meal and snack.
____ Drink power drinks.
____ Practice deep breathing, which nourishes and recharges your system while inducing relaxation and clarity. Indulge in slow, deep breathing all day long, especially before meals.
____ Provide your body with the vitamins, minerals, and other

nutrients you need for repair and to loosen the strangle-hold of your addiction. Your personal program can be found in chapter 9.

___ Do what you can to eliminate white flour and sugar.

___ Avoid processed, junk, and fake foods and/or chemicals.

___ Drink organic green tea, which has half the caffeine of coffee, is filled with antioxidants, and does not contain pesticides—if this small amount of caffeine still keeps you awake, it is best not to drink green tea.

___ Drink detox tea.

___ Practice positive thinking.

___ Have some fun every day.

___ Engage in moderate exercise that you find fun and that clears your mind.

___ Be in sunshine every day if possible.

___ Pray and listen to inspiring music.

Salt

For many years the medical community hypothesized that water retention from excessive amounts of salt raised blood pressure. Doctors have traditionally encouraged their patients to restrict salt. Recent studies have shown that only ten percent of people with high blood pressure are actually salt sensitive. *If you are diabetic, or have been put on a no-salt diet by your doctor, check with your doctor before you make any dietary or supplement changes.*

People with low blood pressure need not restrict salt. Completely avoiding salt can cause the adrenals to hyperfunction in an attempt to make up for the salt deficit. Some people need more salt than others, and by simply providing their body with salt they can correct their insomnia. If you recognize yourself as a salt-restrictor and you suffer from insomnia, adding some salt to your diet is a good place to begin. Those who have restricted salt for a long time may feel a little swollen the first week they add it back to their diet. This will generally pass in three to seven days. By continuing to use salt your body will shift to a better balance and will let go of the fluid retention.

Digestive Problems

Madeline suffers from serious digestive problems stemming from years of insomnia. "For the last few years I've gotten intense pains in my stomach," Madeline said. "I don't know when it's coming, but I always know it's stress related." Her digestive problems do stem from stress—from remaining in a sympathetic-dominant state because of constant worrying and fretting.

All of the systems of the body, such as digestion, reproduction, and immune surveillance, require a very specific pH in which to function. The proper functioning of all the systems of the body, including all of the literally millions of biochemical processes within these systems, depends on a precise system of checks and balances that adjusts your body's pH accordingly.

The digestive tract is a perfect example of the precise system of checks and balances that hinge on the body's correct pH balance. The digestive system is a very orderly system that goes from a pH of 1 to 3.5, which is acid, all the way to a pH of 7 to 8, which is alkaline, by the time food reaches the end of the digestive process and is eliminated. In approximately every one to two feet of our intestines the pH is monitored and regulated by an interactive feedback system between your brain and digestive system.

Your digestive system should not turn on all at once. That would flush food right through you. This would be caused by bacteria (from eating spoiled food or taking harsh laxatives or too much magnesium which is cathartic).

Nor should your digestive system turn off all at once—which would cause any undigested foods to be caught midway in the digestive process and left to rot. This would result in indigestion, bloating, cramping, gas, and constipation. Your digestive system and peristalsis turn off when you are in a state of sympathetic dominance. When your body thinks that you are in danger, for example, running from a tiger in the woods, you do not need to be digesting food. Energy is shunted to the systems that will help you fight or flee or otherwise deal with danger. To your body, constantly worrying and fretting, habitually running late for work, or arguing with your spouse are varying degrees of danger. In fact, any highly charged event or activity—even fun and excitement—will stimulate the adrenaline fight-or-flight response and keep you from digesting food properly.

When digestion is working correctly, the muscles of the digestive tract advance food along the way to break down and assimilate nutrients. When each stage is complete, the muscles of peristalsis—the organized, rhythmic muscular contraction of the digestive tract that moves food from the mouth through the digestive system—push the food along to the next process until elimination. Digestion works properly when you regularly eat a balanced diet of real, whole foods and when you get enough rest along with all the other factors spelled out in the Ten Simple Solutions.

The beginning of your digestive process begins in your mouth with chewing and salivary enzymes, which begin the breakdown of food. At the next stop, stomach acids begin dissolving food and activating protein-digesting enzymes. When food goes from the stomach to the entry of the small intestine, the pancreas releases alkaline fluids and enzymes, which neutralize stomach acid. The partially digested food then progresses through your small intestine, where, now that the acid has been buffered, enzymes can assimilate nutrients without being destroyed. If partially digested food remains too acidic, the enzymes released by your pancreas are damaged by the stomach acid, and your food will be delayed. While the food sits in your stomach and/or small intestine and rots, it may belch back up, a condition known as gastroesophageal reflux disease (GERD), better known as heartburn. Likewise, if the food is held up anywhere along the digestive process, you may experience other types of problems such as indigestion, bloating, cramping, gas, and constipation.

If you remain in a sympathetic-dominant state, the pendulum of your body's autonomic nervous system cannot naturally ebb and flow with the alkaline tide. When your body is too acidic, the pH in your digestive tract cannot be adjusted and digestive problems will occur.

Under-Forty Prescription for Digestive Problems

If you are under forty and suffer from esophageal reflux or gastritis, it could be that your sympathetic nervous system has shut off digestion and your stomach is full of rotting, fermenting food that needs somewhere to go. If your sympathetic nervous system is regularly turning off your digestion, leaving large amounts of food in your stomach, then your stomach may eventually stretch out. The high-tension ring-shaped muscle called the lower esophageal sphincter, which maintains constriction to prevent the stomach's corrosive digestive juices from escaping into the esophagus, will become lax. Your stomach contents, aided by gravity when you lie down, will gurgle up into your esophagus and cause gastroesophageal reflux disease (GERD), or heartburn. Heartburn is a burning sensation under the breastbone that can radiate toward the mouth.

If you suffer from occasional indigestion, take a combination of the following herbs. See page 355 for companies that make digestive herbal formulas.

If you suffer from occasional indigestion, take a formula that contains:

An herbal decoction of poria fungus, Job's tears seed, pueraria root, saussurea root, magnolia bark, patchouli leaf, angelica, dahurica root, atractylodes rhizome, fermented leaven, rice sprouts, chrysanthemum flower, gastrodia rhizome, tangerine peel, peppermint leaf, trichosanthes root.

Or if you are suffering from chronic gastritis or GERD, before meals and at bedtime take a formula that contains deglycyrrhinated licorice root—the glycyrrhinic acid that raises blood pressure in some individuals is removed. It has been shown that licorice root accelerates the actions of the cells that provide a protective coating for the lining of the stomach.

Licorice root has been shown to be comparable to the antacid Tagamet.

One to three times a day, take a formula that contains:

3,500 milligrams L-Glutamine
300 milligrams deglycyrrhinated licorice root
50 milligrams aloe leaf extract
The third dose should be taken at bedtime.

Also take an enzyme formula that contains:

20,000 PC protease I	600 units peptidase
200,000 USP protease II	600 DP maltase
40,000 HUT protease	400 lactase
20,000 LU amylase	400 invertase
2,000 LU lipase	49 milligrams amla fruit
2,000 CU cellulase	

Also:

- Avoid conflict during meals.

- Take five or ten deep breaths before meals.

- Chew your food. There are digestive enzymes in your mouth that are released by chewing, which stimulates the activity of proper stomach digestion.

Over-Forty Prescription for Digestive Problems

If you are over forty and suffering from chronic gastritis or GERD, before meals and at bedtime take a formula that contains deglycyrrhinated licorice root—the glycyrrhinic acid is removed that raises blood pressure in some individuals. It has been shown that licorice root accelerates the actions of the cells that provide a protective coating of the lining of the stomach. Licorice root has been shown to be comparable to the antacid Tagamet.

Three times a day take a formula that contains:

> 3,500 milligrams L-Glutamine
> 300 milligrams deglycyrrhinated licorice root
> 50 milligrams aloe leaf extract
> The third dose should be taken at bedtime.

Also take an enzyme formula that contains:

> 20,000 PC protease I   600 units peptidase
> 200,000 USP protease II   600 DP maltase
> 40,000 HUT protease   400 lactase
> 20,000 LU amylase   400 invertase
> 2,000 LU lipase   49 millgrams amla fruit
> 2,000 CU cellulase

Hydrochloric Acid Supplement Recommendations for Those with Too Little Stomach Acid

Begin with:

> 1 teaspoon to 1 tablespoon apple cider vinegar in water, with your meal

> *If this is not effective, add:* 2 to 10 grains (120 to 600 milligrams) hydrochloric acid (HCl) with food.

> You can buy hydrochloric acid at your health food store.

Also:

- Avoid conflict during meals.

- Take five or ten deep breaths before meals.

- Chew your food. There are digestive enzymes in your mouth that are released by chewing. Chewing stimulates the activity of the proper stomach digestion.

If your system does not make enough hydrochloric acid, the food will not be able to leave the stomach. Trapped food will sit in your stomach or upper small intestine and rot—a situation that can go on for hours and hours, causing indigestion, bloating, cramping, gas, and constipation. All of this will interfere with your ability to sleep.

It has always been assumed that digestive problems are caused by too much stomach acid. Sometimes it can be just the opposite. As you get older, your digestive system also ages and slows down. Your body may not make enough stomach acid. Because there is not always an easy way to determine if you are the first case or the second case I described, I always encourage people—no matter what their age—to begin with the under-forty prescription first, and if that does not work to switch to the over-forty prescription.

Taking a hydrochloric acid supplement turns on digestion and peristalsis. But if your stomach is already raw, too much stomach acid will make you uncomfortable for an hour or two. If this occurs, drink one or two glasses of water.

Acupressure

There are acupressure points on the bottom of the feet that help digestion. A great way to massage these points is to take a tennis ball and step lightly onto it, rolling it around under your foot, including your instep. This is a well-known reflex point that opens up the exit path for food to move out of your stomach.

Music

In recent years, the healing effects of music, in particular the music of Mozart, have been brought to the attention of the medical community. Many studies have been done on the effects of music on creativity, learning, health, and healing. The calming effects of music on the nervous system are well documented. Half an hour of music has been shown to produce the same effect as ten milligrams of Valium.

In a study at the Miami Veterans Administration Medical Center, involving twenty male patients with Alzheimer's disease, thirty- to forty-minute morning sessions of music therapy five times per week for four weeks significantly increased the concentration of the sleep hormone melatonin in patients' bloodstreams. The patients' melatonin levels were found to increase even further at a six-week follow-up visit. The patients' increased levels of melatonin following music therapy contributed to more relaxed and calmer moods.

The music that you listen to all day and at night will make it easier or harder to sleep. Your nervous system is stimulated or calmed by the music. If you listen to anything but soothing music, you will overstimulate your nervous system. A study on the effects of rock music, researchers found that university students who were exposed to music by the Beatles, Jimi Hendrix, the Rolling Stones, Led Zeppelin, and music from other bands of that ilk breathed faster and had an increased heart rate compared to those exposed to random background noise. Recommendations for music and relaxation tapes begin on page 350.

Unwanted Noise

Noise pollution is a ubiquitous problem of our times. Whether we know it or not, every noise is channeled into the production of your neurotransmitters.

A study on noise annoyance in the intensive care unit (ICU) demonstrated that music intervention with cardiac surgery patients during the first postoperative day decreased noise annoyance, thereby decreasing heart rate and blood pressure. If you cannot sleep because of your neighbors' barking dogs or TVs or the sounds of nearby traffic, music can be calming and soothing and can help mask unwanted background noise and soothe your nerves.

There are also white noise machines that can deflect unwanted sounds and mask discordant noise—even snoring—which will allow you to get to sleep. There are a number of quality sleeping machines available that are about the size of a clock radio. White noise machines mask unwanted noise by producing a smooth sound of rushing air to create a sense of calm. Others produce a variety of low-frequency digital sounds, including the sounds of a lakeshore, rain, surf, a brook, a waterfall, and a "country evening." These types of sounds have been repeatedly proven to lower heart rate and motor activity and induce sleep. Another machine, which provides womb, heartbeat, and lullaby sounds, was developed specifically for infants and small children, but adults can enjoy it as well. Product recommendations can be found on page 356.

Madeline has begun taking the sleep formula and has been incorporating other positive habits into her life such as deep breathing and positive thinking. She is beginning to see results. "In just a couple of weeks I've noticed a big difference," she said. "When I wake up in the middle of the night, I'm not wide-awake. I feel sleepy, and I've been able to get back to sleep." Together with the sleep supplements and other techniques, Madeline will eventually conquer her lifelong insomnia. As her body restores her adrenal reserve, the other systems of her body will begin to function more smoothly, and she will see her overall health improve.

Night owls

We have covered several important factors that contribute to insomnia. We have not yet talked about night owls: the segment of the population who are biologically night people. Now that we are beginning to do saliva testing in the middle of the night, we may find that many night owls have high cortisol, which indicates that their rhythm is different from the day person. It is important for night people to work with their rhythm.

You know you are a night person if

___ you read under the covers when you were little
___ you hated getting up in the morning, and you still hate it
___ you are grouchy and uncommunicative in the morning

___ you are creative and productive after the sun goes down

___ you love to stay up half the night or even all night

If you recognize that you are a night person, do what you can to live peacefully with your rhythm. If you are more productive and happier when you stay up late at night and sleep in past what day people see as an acceptable hour, make peace with yourself about it. If possible, find a career that allows you to be creative and productive during your peak hours. The computer age has allowed many companies to shift from bricks and mortar to virtual offices. Working at home on your own schedule may be the best solution for you. If you marry a day person, which you probably will, do what you can to work out a comfortable arrangement.

Unfortunately, our world often demands that we be productive at all hours of the day and night, which deters us from our innate rhythm. Any time that you are out of your natural rhythm, your body is stressed.

Whether it is doing yoga, listening to peaceful music, going for a gentle stroll, being in nature, or finding a new job, anything you can do to bring yourself back to your natural rhythm will help your body work better. And anything you can do to get your body back into harmony with itself will help repair your fatigue, your health, and your vitality.

Simple Solution 4: Pay off Your Sleep Debt
Tailored to your stage of burnout

Driven and Dragging

___ If you are Driven, you need six to eight hours of sleep every night—even if you think you can get away with less. If you are Dragging, you need eight hours.

___ Thinking positive thoughts about sleep will continue to produce healthy neurotransmitters, which will prevent you from developing insomnia in the future.

___ Cultivate healthy sleep habits now before you develop sleep problems.

___ Stop eating sugar at night now before you develop sleep problems. Eat protein instead.

___ Quit caffeine now before it has a firm grip on you and before you develop sleep problems. Wean off coffee gently.

___ Nap as needed—go ahead and indulge yourself.

___ When you get home from work or school, listen to relaxing music to begin to condition your mind that home is a time for relaxing. See pages 350–352 for recommendations.

Losing It and Hitting the Wall

___ Eight hours of sleep every night is critical if you are Losing It. If you are Hitting the Wall, eight to nine hours is your prescription.

___ More often than not, your sleep is disrupted now. To restore adrenal reserves, it is more important than ever for you to get a good night's rest every night. Begin by thinking positive thoughts about sleep to produce healthy neurotransmitters, which will aid in making you drowsy and sleepy.

___ Decide what you can do to change your habits now before your insomnia gets firmly entrenched. You will thank yourself later on.

___ Two ten-to-fifteen-minute quiet retreat periods per day is the minimum, such as going for a walk or closing your eyes for ten minutes. Go into the restroom, close the door, and rest or meditate there if you cannot find another private place.

___ Learn to associate your bedroom with sleep. Make your bedroom your sanctuary.

___ Positive exercises and supplements can neutralize disruptive thoughts that keep you awake obsessing.

___ Eating sugar at night will keep you awake and add even more unwanted pounds at this stage. If you are hungry, try

the "Grandmother Method," a bedtime snack of protein, especially turkey, cottage cheese or organic, raw milk, which
will provide your body with the calming neurotransmitter
tryptophan.

___ Quit caffeine—but not cold turkey. Wean off coffee gently
with the help of the serotonin-boosting guidelines provided
on page 172 and the recommended supplements for your
stage of burnout.

___ Listen to relaxing music when you get home from work.
Positive imagery tapes can help lull you to sleep at night and
help create those calming neurotransmitters that will make
you a healthier more positive person. See pages 350–352 for
recommendations.

___ If noise is keeping you awake and there is nothing you can
do about it, consider using a white noise machine. See page
356 for product recommendations.

Burned Out

___ Sleep is your number-one priority now that you are burned
out. At this stage, your health is in a delicate balance. If at all
possible, take a leave of absence, go on disability, or at most,
work part time.

___ Eight to ten hours of sleep every night is critical.

___ Fifteen-to-thirty minutes restful retreats are in order—three
times a day, napping in a serene environment.

___ Think positive thoughts about sleep to produce healthy
neurotransmitters, which will aid in making you drowsy and
sleepy.

___ Now that you have the time to cultivate healthy sleep habits,
baby yourself.

___ You have a good excuse now to go to bed early. Even on the
days when you feel more energetic, avoid staying up late
and doing agitating activities that will make it impossible to
sleep.

___ You need a sanctuary now more than ever. Take the phone and TV out of your bedroom. Learn to associate your bedroom with sleep.

___ Practice positive exercises and supplements to neutralize disruptive thoughts that keep you awake obsessing.

___ If you are kept awake by muscle spasms, take magnesium supplements.

___ Eating sugar at night now is one of the worst habits you can have. You do need a snack at bedtime, so try the "Grandmother Method," a snack of protein, especially turkey, cottage cheese or organic, raw milk, which will provide your body with the calming neurotransmitter tryptophan.

___ Quitting caffeine is crucial now. Do not go cold turkey—this will be too much of a shock on your already worn out adrenals. Wean off coffee gently with the help of the serotonin-boosting guidelines on page 172 and the recommended supplements for your stage of burnout.

___ If you are a salt-restrictor, and you suffer from insomnia, add some salt to your diet (with your doctor's permission).

___ If gastrointestinal problems are causing your insomnia, take the digestive formulas provided on pages 176–179.

___ Listening to relaxing music during the day and positive imagery tapes at bedtime will keep you in a calm state. See pages 350–352 for recommendations.

___ If noise is keeping you awake, you are ill and have every right to ask your neighbors for consideration. Explain your situation and see if dogs and children can be quieted. If you cannot do anything about the noise, purchase a white noise machine. See page 356 for product recommendations.

8

Simple Solution 5
Let Go of Your
Favorite Poison

*Sugar, stimulants, and drugs
are wolves in sheep's clothing*

Shortcuts to Simple Solution 5

- Say good-bye to stimulants such as sugar, caffeine, nicotine, ma huang, guarana, and ephedra.

- Use serotonin boosting formulas to kick the stimulant habit.

Fifty-two-year-old Rachel Kantor lives in a brand new townhouse on what was the epicenter of the devastating 1994 Northridge earthquake. It is a metaphor for the time bomb she once carried around inside her. Rachel, who does not have an ounce of fat on her body, explained that her lifelong philosophy was to "stay close to the bone," a quote she attributed to Jane Fonda. "I had this poster from the Schwarzenegger movie *Stay Hungry*," she explained. "It was like you needed the edge. If you sat down and had a full meal then you didn't have your edge anymore. The way to have your edge is to actually look like an edge. So that was my ideal."

When Rachel called my office she was asked in advance of her appointment to write down everything she ate for a week. Rachel was shocked when she saw her diet in black and white. "Everything that I ate had sugar in it," she said. "In the morning I would have a croissant and a cappuccino with four teaspoons of sugar. I ate M & Ms or Godiva chocolates at night." Rachel had reached the Hitting the Wall stage and was dangerously close to being Burned Out.

Sugar

Sugar is the most commonly used stimulant. Sugar is a white, refined, crystalline substance that affects your moods and your behavior. It makes you want more and leaves you cranky when you do not have it. Sugar consumption depletes B vitamins and lowers your body's resistance to bacteria, viruses, and yeasts. Sugar makes your brain irritable and hyperactive.

Regardless of your sugar form of choice—whether it is bagels, cookies, pies, candy, pasta, rice cakes, sodas, fruit juice, white, raw, or brown sugar, fructose, corn syrup, or honey—all sugar leads to the adrenaline/cortisol/insulin vicious cycle that will put you on a blood sugar roller coaster and ultimately deplete your adrenal reserve.

When you eat sugar it enters your bloodstream all at once, instead of slowly as it would as part of real, whole foods. Insulin is secreted and stores that sugar away into cells. Now that there is not enough sugar in your bloodstream, your brain senses that you are in a time of famine and sends a red alert to your adrenals to release adrenaline and cortisol. Adrenaline releases energy from sugar stored in your liver and muscles, and cortisol *breaks down your own muscle mass* to turn it into sugar. Since excess sugar damages brain and body cells—as in diabetes—this influx of sugar into your bloodstream triggers the secretion of insulin, which immediately stores away this new sugar into cells.

This breaking-down and storing-away of sugar will recur again and again as long as you continue to eat sugar and other refined carbohydrates. If you are in the habit of eating sugar, day after day, your adrenals will be continually responding to red alerts from your brain and secreting adrenaline and cortisol to manage your blood sugar. Eventually your adrenal reserve will become depleted, and you will suffer from decreased muscle mass, fat around your middle, a flabby body, hypoglycemia, lowered metabolism, premature accelerated aging, and even type II diabetes.

If that were not bad enough, eating sugar also causes the insulin/serotonin vicious cycle that causes cravings, mood swings, and depression.

Serotonin, known as the feel-good neurotransmitter, is made from, among other nutrients, the amino acid tryptophan, found in protein. When you eat protein, your body produces serotonin. Some is used immediately, and the rest is stored in a reservoir in your brain. When you eat sugar, the actions of insulin facilitate the entry of tryptophan into your brain. It is not known exactly how, but this passage of tryptophan causes the release of serotonin from the reservoir in your brain. This is why eating sugar makes you feel good.

When you eat a sugar diet and do not eat the protein precursors to serotonin, your brain will crave sugar. Eating sugar will cause the release of serotonin from the storage reservoir in your brain. If you continue to eat sugar, your body and brain will be trapped in these two vicious cycles. Eventually your storage reservoir of serotonin will begin to run dry, and there will come a time when there is a negligible amount of serotonin to release. No matter how much sugar you eat, you will not get that feel-good serotonin response. At this point, people often eat even more sugar, especially at night, and eventually turn to antidepressants.

Eating sugar at night causes

Acne	Mood swings and PMS
Extreme fatigue	Weight gain, especially
Increased colds and flu	around the middle
Insomnia	Yeast infections
Irritability	

Figure 6
The Vicious Cycles

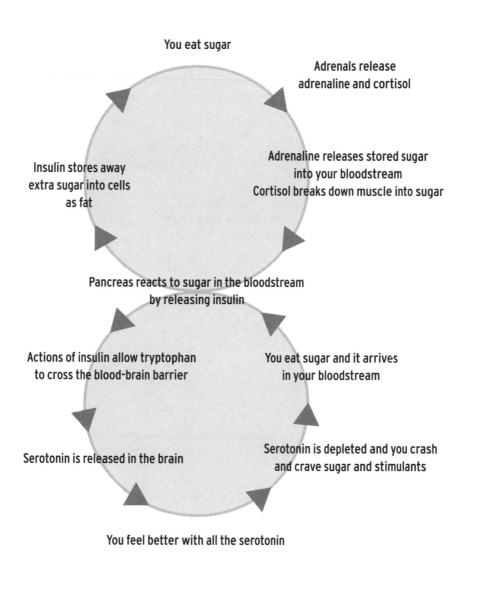

You eat sugar

Adrenals release
adrenaline and cortisol

Insulin stores away
extra sugar into cells
as fat

Adrenaline releases stored sugar
into your bloodstream
Cortisol breaks down muscle into sugar

Pancreas reacts to sugar in the bloodstream
by releasing insulin

Actions of insulin allow tryptophan
to cross the blood-brain barrier

You eat sugar and it arrives
in your bloodstream

Serotonin is released in the brain

Serotonin is depleted and you crash
and crave sugar and stimulants

You feel better with all the serotonin

These two vicious cycles working simultaneously result in both a blood sugar roller coaster and a serotonin roller coaster. Your adrenals are futilely working overtime to stabilize both situations. Eventually your adrenal reserve will be depleted.

The adrenaline/cortisol/insulin vicious cycle puts you on a blood sugar roller coaster that causes:

Decreased muscle mass   Hypoglycemia
Lowered metabolism   Premature aging
Fat around your middle   Type II diabetes
Flabby body

The insulin/serotonin vicious cycle puts you on a mood swing roller coaster that causes:

Anxiety   Insomnia
Cravings   Irritability
Crying jags   Mood swings
Depression

Figure 7
Roller-coaster cravings

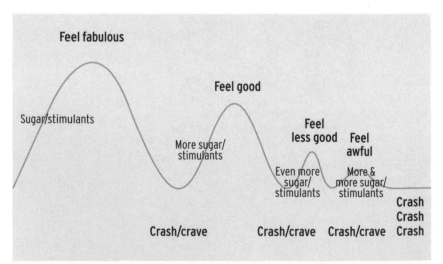

Even though Rachel suffered from mood swings she was resistant to the idea of giving up sugar. "Doctor Hanley said that I most likely had the blood sugar level of a diabetic. I told her, 'Listen, my way of eating has worked for me all of these years.' Doctor Hanley looked me in the eye and said, 'Rachel, it's payback time.'"

I wanted to get Rachel's attention because I was certain that a blood panel would confirm that she was dangerously close to developing type II diabetes, also known as adult onset diabetes. When people eat a lot of sugar, their glucose (blood sugar) is consistently high and a candy coating builds up on their cells and arteries, called glycosylation (*gly ko si lay shun*). Glycosylation gets in the way of metabolic processes. Nutrients cannot get into the candy-coated cells, and worse, trash cannot get out. Rachel's tests told me that at the time her blood was drawn she was hypoglycemic, which was to be expected considering her high-sugar diet.

Hypoglycemia is caused by eating too much sugar, including fruit, fruit juices, and refined carbohydrates and grains, and/or by not eating for long periods of time. When you eat sugar, an immediate insulin response goes to work, stowing the dangerous excess sugar safely away into cells. This sudden blood sugar crash is known as hypoglycemia. Hypoglycemia, or low blood sugar, occurs when blood sugar levels dip too fast and too low.

A hypoglycemic emergency is like getting on an airplane with only enough fuel to get halfway to your destination. When the fuel tanks run dry, the plane starts to fall out of the sky until the pilot can get the emergency stores of fuel to switch in, and then all of a sudden the plane starts to fly again—until it begins to sputter and nosedive once again. It is a terrifying experience for the people on the plane. Likewise, when your blood sugar drops, you can become foggy, irritable, and incoherent. You can see spots in front of your eyes, get shaky, become dizzy, and even become unconscious.

In addition to her hypoglycemia, Rachel's tests also told me that she was on a clear course toward developing type II diabetes. One of insulin's jobs is to stow away sugar and nutrients into your cells for use or for storage. Cells contain a certain number of doors that are called insulin receptors. These doors can only be opened when insulin stimulates the door's receptors. The secretion of insulin is stimulated by eating carbohydrates. If insulin is high in your bloodstream over a prolonged period of time, your cell's insulin receptors become desensitized to the actions of insulin and lose their ability to respond. Insulin can no longer deposit as much sugar and nutrients into cells. This condition is called insulin resistance. When a person is insulin resistant and continues to eat too much sugar, the pancreas secretes even *more* insulin in an attempt to force the receptors to respond. Now there is too much insulin in the bloodstream, a condition known as hyperinsulinemia (*hi per in sue lin ee mia*), a precursor to type II diabetes and a risk factor for cardiac heart disease. Your hyperinsulinemic cells become even less responsive to insulin. As the cells become increasingly desensitized, more and more sugar remains in the bloodstream, a condition known as type II diabetes.

Recent reports indicate that Americans are experiencing an epidemic of type II diabetes. Although type II diabetes usually strikes after age forty, between 1990 and 1998 there was an overall 30 percent increase in the number of cases of type II diabetes diagnosed and a 76 percent increase in people in their *thirties*. Medical science has long known that diabetes is firmly linked to obesity. The percentage of obese Americans, defined as 30 pounds or more overweight, has increased from 12 percent in 1991 to 21 percent in 2000 and is still climbing. In the last decades the incidence of type II diabetes has risen in all major ethnic groups.

Eating too much sugar or too many refined-flour products can also lead to heart disease. For over forty years studies have demonstrated that prolonged high insulin levels cause hypertension, high cholesterol (high triglycerides, high LDLs—the bad cholesterol), and atheroslerosis (plaquing of the arteries), which significantly contribute to heart attack and stroke.

Rachel's father died of a stroke when he was seventy-three from complications of diabetes. "When Doctor Hanley talked to me, I remembered the harrowing months when my father was struggling for his life. I just thought to myself that death as a lifestyle wouldn't work for me. Especially dying slowly and painfully. I have a daughter who was twelve then, and thinking that I wasn't going to be there for her terrified me. So I went home and gave up everything that had sugar in it. Doctor Hanley said that she wasn't going to ask me to give up coffee because she wanted me to come back. But since I only like coffee if it tastes like a malted, I gave up coffee too."

Unwittingly, we are all driven by our psychogenes, which lead us down long winding roads that often end up in behaviors such as eating too much sugar. Rachel believed that money and status equaled happiness, and her fear that she would be unhappy without them → led to fear of failure → led to overwork and not eating → led to inability to keep going, financial ruin, and ultimately depression. As Rachel said, part of her belief system was that "you needed the edge. If you sat down and had a full meal then you didn't have your edge anymore." Rachel intentionally withheld food from herself because of a misguided belief that it would give her more of an edge to be successful. She ended up craving and living on sugar.

Whatever your psychogene, you may feel that you do not have time to eat, and this may have driven you to rely on quick fixes of sugar, craving and even living on sugar. When you eat regularly you are not constantly hungry, and your cravings for sweets disappear. Instead of your mind driving you in panic and desperation for a quick fix, you can make better food choices. By nourishing your body with regular balanced meals of real, whole food you will gain your edge to be more successful. You will have more stamina, more of an optimistic attitude about yourself and life, and more ability to deal with life's issues with self-confidence.

Rachel, who was in the Hitting the Wall stage, narrowly avoided type II diabetes. By giving up sugar and eating regular balanced meals of real, whole foods, she got off the blood sugar roller coaster that had been running her ragged for many years with cravings and mood swings. Rachel has had normal blood sugar levels for over two years now and feels the best she has in her adult life and has the most energy.

If you are interested in seeing how much sugar you eat, keep a sugar journal for one week. Make photocopies of these pages or write in a journal. Keep in mind that many products, especially condiments, contain sugar. Be sure to check labels carefully. You will be surprised to see how much sugar is in processed foods.

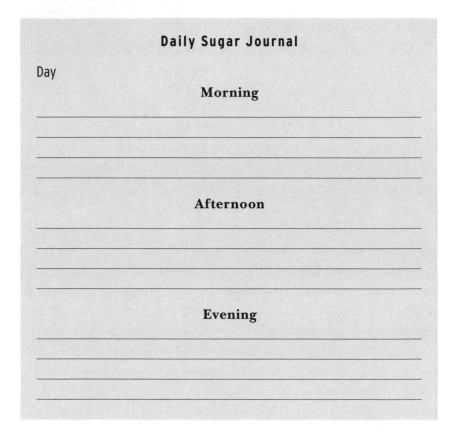

Daily Sugar Journal

Day

Morning

Afternoon

Evening

People learn to overeat carbohydrates, particularly comfort foods such as chips, ice cream, candy, popcorn, and cereal from enticing advertising, family customs, and their own pleasurable experiences. If you want to get off the sugar-craving roller coaster, the single most important factor in conquering sugar cravings is to eat small meals and snacks that contain protein, fat, and some carbohydrate. *Avoid refined carbohydrates.* Eat six balanced meals of real, whole food a day—three meals and three snacks. Please turn to pages 206–207 the end of this chapter for formulas to boost serotonin and help you defeat your sugar cravings.

. . .

There are not many safe alternatives to white sugar. Molasses and unrefined honey are better choices than refined white sugar because they both contain a healthy array of nutrients, so their cost to our health is not as severe as that of white sugar. Brown sugar and turbinado masquerade as healthy sugars but are really no better than refined white sugar. *Never consume aspartame and saccharin.* If you have to have your sugar fix, here are some healthy alternatives to sugar.

Crystallized Raw Cane Juice

This raw sugar contains chromium and other nutrient complexes that cause it to be absorbed slowly so it does not result in as rapid an insulin release as white sugar. This is my favorite sugar substitute because it is a whole food. Studies show that crystallized raw cane juice does not contribute to cavities, insulin resistance, or type II diabetes.

Stevia

Known as "honey leaf," stevia is made from a South American herb. It is two hundred times sweeter than refined white sugar but does not trigger an insulin response, so it is safe to eat. Stevia has an unpleasant aftertaste to some. Many feel it is worth putting up with the taste for the sake of having something sweet to eat. Many people actually grow to like it.

Xylitol

Extracted from birch trees, xylitol looks and tastes like refined white sugar. It is not carbohydrate free, but clinical trials have shown that it is metabolized slowly, so it stimulates slower insulin release. Xylitol changes the bacterial makeup in the mouth and eliminates cavity-causing pathogens.

Sorbitol

Made from Jerusalem artichokes, sorbitol is a healthy and safe sugar substitute.

Fructooligosaccharides
(fruk toe ola go saka rides) (FOS)

A sweetener commonly used in Japan, FOS is derived from various roots that have beneficial effects as food ingredients. FOS is absorbed slowly and minimally in the digestive tract so it does not cause a rapid insulin release. FOS is known to promote, stabilize, and enhance the proliferation of probiotics, such as acidophilus, bifidus, and faecium, which are beneficial intestinal bacteria.

You can buy any of these healthy sugars in your virtual or bricks-and-mortar health food store.

Caffeine

Thirty-three-year-old Caitlin Takahashi is a rep for a film production company in Manhattan. She was working sixty to seventy hours per week. In addition to her work schedule, for several months she had been driving four hours round trip on the weekends to Philadelphia to sit at the bedside of a friend who was dying. Caitlin was feeling the effects of the fatigue and stress. "One Saturday, I woke up early in the morning, drove to Philadelphia and spent the day there," she remembered. "I left at 4 P.M., drove back to Manhattan, dropped off a friend, and kept going out to Long Island. I had to drive another two hours to get to a party for an important client. I had wine with dinner. Then I realized I needed a clear head to get back to the city, so I started pounding down heavy-duty French roast coffee. I lost track of how many cups I drank. I arrived back in the city after midnight. When I lay down to sleep it was like a bomb went off in my body. My heart rate soared. I was freezing cold and sweating and felt like I was going to pass out. I called my cousin, who is a doctor, and he called an ambulance. At the hospital, he and the attending physician told me I was suffering from caffeine intoxication." The second most commonly used stimulant is caffeine—an odorless, slightly bitter alkaloid found in coffee, tea, chocolate, sodas, and some medications. Many people use caffeine indiscriminately, and others just do not realize the harmful effects. Either way, it is important for you to realize how the caffeine in your sodas and coffee add up during the day and can result in the caffeine intoxication Caitlin experienced. Excessive intake of caffeine can cause restlessness, insomnia, heart irregularities, panic attacks, and even delirium.

Regular caffeine intake increases cortisol levels and lowers DHEA levels, which eventually depletes your adrenal reserve. While it is appropriate and necessary to be in a sympathetic-dominant state part of the time, using stimulants such as caffeine keeps your body too acidic and in a constant state of sympathetic dominance. These behaviors cause your adrenals to pump continually, which ultimately depletes your adrenal reserve, leading to weight gain, chronic conditions, illnesses, and disease.

I never ask people to quit caffeine cold turkey. If you have been squeezing the life out of your adrenals by drinking coffee, if you stop drinking coffee abruptly, the demand on your exhausted adrenals stops suddenly. Since it takes time for your adrenals to recover enough to begin to respond to nonemergency demand, you may feel weak, headachy, fatigued and nauseated and have cravings. Back off from coffee gently, follow the serotonin-boosting formula on page 206 for quitting addictions, and take the supplements recommended in Chapter 9 for your stage of burnout.

Your craving will gradually diminish. Your adrenals will repair and begin to respond again. Weaning yourself off coffee slowly will allow you to feel better along the way, instead of suffering from withdrawal symptoms. Begin by giving up one-half cup of coffee every few days. If you drink three cups of coffee a day, then you can quit in two to three weeks. If you drink ten cups, it may take you up to two months to quit entirely.

Switching to decaffeinated coffee is not the same as quitting, since decaffeinated coffee still contains some and even significant amounts of caffeine. In addition, except for Swiss water-processed decaffeinated coffee, most coffees are decaffeinated with methylene chloride, a carcinogen that you then ingest with your decreased caffeine.

I also encourage you to ask less of yourself during this healing time. Realize that there is a repair process going on. Quitting an addiction like caffeine is a process in which you must be gentle with yourself.

Nicotine

Nicotine, in the form of cigarettes, cigars, and chewing tobacco, Nicotrol, Nicoderm, and other cigarette substitutes, is another socially acceptable, highly abused stimulant. Nicotine is known to cause vascular disease and cancer. Patches, chewing gum, and other products containing nicotine that are advertised to help people kick the nicotine habit are nicotine delivery devices. These products are just as addicting as tobacco products—and many people have traded in one dangerous, expensive habit for another.

It has been said that quitting nicotine is harder than quitting heroin. We have all seen footage of cancer victims smoking out of tracheal tubes in their necks. We know that nicotine's grip is deadly. If you are trying to quit smoking, please be kind to yourself during this healing time. Realize that there is a repair process going on that takes time, and you will feel better with each passing week. Today there is no reason to quit alone. Consider seeking professional help or quit with a little help from a *real* friend, not another nicotine product.

Herbal Stimulants

Forty-five-year-old Jacqueline Clark is a leggy, tanned, and attractive blonde—the very picture of someone who would own and run a modeling agency in Hollywood. She is able to make whomever she is addressing feel special and singled out. She is also breathlessly intense—a reflection of her high-energy lifestyle. "I erected a demanding business," Jacqueline began. "It was really like operating several businesses at the same time. It was a finishing school, a photography studio, and an agency. I run every one of the facets of my businesses to perfection. My clients are important to me, and nothing is too good for them. I want every one of them to be successful, and I take things much too personally. When my business needs something done, I will stay until midnight until it gets done. I'm a perfectionist when it comes to raising my three children too. So for years and years I have been on the go too much and have pushed too much and have tried to do too much every day." Jacqueline was on the track toward burnout.

A year and a half ago, she began suffering from anxiety and irregular heartbeats. "Prior to that, to lose weight, I was taking an herbal product that contained [the herbal stimulants] ephedra and ma huang," Jacqueline said. "I would get a buzz from it, and it did help me lose weight. I would feel great—ecstatic and euphoric. But it also made my heartbeat a little irregular."

All stimulants, including natural stimulants, are referred to as sympathomimetic (*sim path o mim et ick*), that is, they mimic and magnify the actions of adrenaline. Stimulants rev cellular functions: you think faster; your heart beats faster; your body creates and burns energy faster. Stimulants also make the body more acidic and cause you to be a state of sympathetic dominance.

For many people the hyped-up feeling from using stimulants is exhilarating. They get hooked on the temporary good feelings and energy they get from using stimulants. Being on stimulants is like being on an extreme adrenaline rush. The duration will vary, depending on the stimulant and a person's body size and composition. Nonetheless, because your body is not meant to be in a constant state of sympathetic overdrive, everyone who uses stimulants will eventually begin to feel agitated and anxious sooner or later. Your thoughts will become jumbled. Your behavior will become clipped and darting. Although most people do not enjoy the pounding heart and jittery nerves, they get hooked on stimulants by the initial good feelings and keep going back for more. People in the later stages of burnout increasingly reach for stimulants and drugs in a vain attempt to recreate a temporary boost of energy and a momentary lift in mood that once came naturally.

Stimulants stress your body and lead to adrenal disaster both by causing the release of adrenaline and by mimicking and exaggerating the actions of adrenaline. This eventually results in depleting your adrenal reserve, which will lead to anxiety, mood swings, and insomnia. In addition to damaging your adrenals, using stimulants also taxes and depletes your body's balancing and calming neurotransmitters, which creates the potential for panic attacks. "I started having some horrible anxiety symptoms from the herbal diet pills," Jacqueline explained. "I felt like I was going to pass out. I felt like I was going to die. I knew that something was really wrong. I had strong feelings of 'uncomfortableness' that I can't really describe. I just wanted it to go away. I remember telling my husband where I had put some jewelry because at one point I really thought I was going to die."

Natural stimulants such as ma huang, guarana, and ephedra cannot be used with impunity just because they are natural. All stimulants ultimately result in what I call panic biochemistry when taken long enough. The state of sympathetic dominance is made more extreme by the use of stimulants, because stimulants rapidly use up your calming neurotransmitters. Your calming neurotransmitters keep you at an even keel. As these neurotransmitters are depleted, you can become agitated and are more easily pushed over the edge. Every little thing becomes a big deal. This is exactly what was happening to Jacqueline. "My anxiety got so bad that I started having nausea and actually throwing up," Jacqueline said. "I got brave enough to go to New York to see an anxiety specialist I had heard about. I wasn't even sure if I could handle the plane ride. In fact, I took a baggie with me because I just didn't want to be in a parking lot or somewhere in an airport and have to throw up and not be able to get to a rest room. That is how sick I was feeling."

Figure 8
Panic Biochemistry

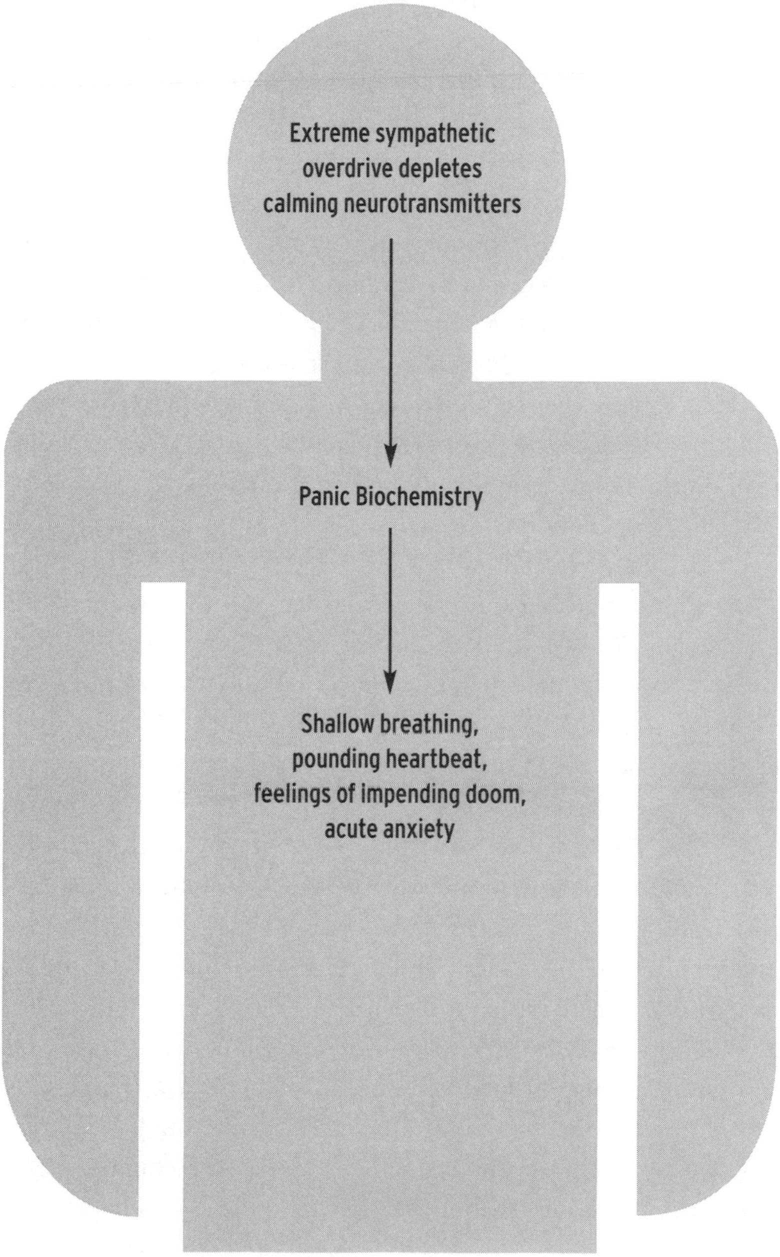

Extreme sympathetic
overdrive depletes
calming neurotransmitters

Panic Biochemistry

Shallow breathing,
pounding heartbeat,
feelings of impending doom,
acute anxiety

Tranquilizers and Antidepressants

The anxiety specialist Jacqueline flew across the country to see prescribed Zanax for her to take during the day to calm her anxiety and Clonopin for her to take at night to help her sleep. Prescription tranquilizers such as Ativan, Clonopin, Valium, Zanax, stimulants such as Cylert, Dexedrine, Fastin, Phentermine, Ritalin, Tenuate, and antidepressants such as Celexa, Paxil, Prozac, Wellbutrin, and Zoloft are the Mother's Little Helpers of the twenty-first century. I could triple this list, but I think you have the idea. Drugs have their place, of course. There are times when it is okay to take medicines as an emergency measure until you can determine a long-term solution. But no matter what your health issue, it is dangerous to think that taking drugs, especially stimulant drugs, are the answer for life. Drugs will eventually deplete healthy neurotransmitters by forcing your body to use them at an accelerated pace. Drugs cause side effects, resulting in deeper depression. You are likely to have a much harder time getting off your drugs the longer you stay on them, and you will be more depleted than when you started.

Jacqueline followed her doctor's advice and took the tranquilizers Zanax and Clonopin. "After feeling better for several months, he also prescribed Tenuate [a prescription stimulant/diet pill] for fatigue and to help me lose weight," Jacqueline said. "I was amazed at what the Tenuate did. It gave me a burst of energy. I felt fabulous. It reminded me of how some diet pills that I had taken in the past had worked. You feel like you can clean your house in five minutes. I loved it and I did lose some weight very slowly. But a couple of months later I started to feel anxious, just like I felt before. There was a lot of tightness in my head. I would ask my husband to give me scalp massages because the top of my head would feel so tight. Then I started getting tired. It got so bad I wondered if it was chronic fatigue syndrome. The anxiety specialist said I should up my Tenuate, but I was afraid to do that. So I called Doctor Hanley instead."

When Jacqueline came to see me, she was suffering from classic Burned Out symptoms: weight gain, exhaustion, and anxiety that had

evolved into panic attacks. Although I encouraged her to wean herself slowly off Tenuate, since Jacqueline is an all-or-nothing person,
she quit Tenuate cold turkey. "I waited twelve days and then I called
Doctor Hanley and told her about how awful I felt, and she said to me
that I was in withdrawal," Jacqueline said. In addition, without the
stimulating effects of Tenuate, Jacqueline was feeling the true exhaustion of her condition. Burned Out is not a state that you can per-
manently mask with drugs. It is a condition that requires a healing
process to fully recover from.

"I started to take three short naps a day and to take the supplements Doctor Hanley prescribed," Jacqueline said. "In just a few days
I could not believe how much better I felt. I started weaning myself
off of Zanax and Clonopin too. After six weeks I felt like my energy
was back. I now have the feeling of well-being and happiness that I
was accustomed to feeling in my life." Jacqueline has since begun to
lose body fat. She has added to her daily supplement formula an oral
spray of homeopathic human growth hormone (hGH) that I recommended, and she feels the best she has in years.

HGH helps balance all the other systems in our body and is the
most potent longevity hormone known. The natural decline of human growth hormone often parallels aging and burnout. The replacement of hGH secretion has been observed to regenerate and
repair most body systems, including adrenals.

One of my patients, Richard Kantor, who had been in on the track
toward burnout for four decades as a highly ambitious clothing manufacturer, began using hGH in conjunction with changing his diet. "I
started using an oral spray of hGH," he said. "Within six months, my
hair, which was as white as snow, is now turning black. I had a receding
hairline, and every month my hairline grew down another half an
inch lower on my forehead. My eyes, which were hazel when I was a
kid and had generally gotten brown through my adult years, have now
turned back to hazel." I cannot guarantee these specific results. I can
only say that hGH is presently the premiere antiaging strategy and
considered by some to be the fountain of youth. In the small doses
that I recommend there are no known adverse side effects.

Selective Serotonin Reuptake Inhibitors (SSRIs)

Although Jacqueline was prescribed tranquilizers and stimulants, many people with her symptoms end up being prescribed selective serotonin reuptake inhibitors (SSRIs) such as Prozac and Zoloft. The recent stampede to SSRIs is one major indication of how burned out our society has become. Unfortunately, SSRIs are not the real solution.

Serotonin is a neurotransmitter that provides an inner sense of well-being and relaxation and promotes restful sleep. For some people, serotonin quiets their obsessive thoughts. When serotonin is high, we feel happy. When it is low, we feel insecure, anxious, depressed, and fearful.

Normal Serotonin Effects

Joy, happiness	Healthy sex drive
Feelings of well-being and peace	Healthy attitudes toward eating
Optimistic attitude about life	Fun-loving
Creativity	Deep, restful sleep
Healthy self-esteem	Energetic

Low Serotonin Effects

Depression, sadness	Stimulant and sugar cravings
Insecurity	Violent and antisocial behavior
Pessimistic attitude about life	
Irritability/anger/rage	Insomnia
Low self-esteem	Headaches and other aches and pains
Low sex drive	

When you provide your body with the proper building blocks of nutrition, serotonin is produced and released in your brain. Some of it is used up, and some of it is reabsorbed in the brain and broken down. In a healthy body, ongoing serotonin production will replace serotonin as it is used up and/or broken down.

SSRIs inhibits the reabsorbtion of serotonin in the brain. With SSRIs, serotonin stays longer in your brain and prolongs the feeling of well-being. If you provide your body with enough protein, which is the precursor to serotonin, SSRIs would continue to work. But since SSRIs do not make serotonin, when serotonin reserves are used up, these drugs cannot help you. In other words, without providing your body with the precursors to make serotonin, eventually—no matter how much SSRI you take—there is little serotonin left in the storage reservoir for the SSRI to work on. This is called SSRI burnout.

Like Jacqueline, Burned Out people are switching to other classes of drugs when SSRIs or their other drugs stop working. Or they add more drugs to the mix. Most people have better options than SSRIs or other drugs to fight emotional difficulties. In fact, the pleasurable feelings you get from the actions of these drugs can be obtained by giving your body protein to restore normal serotonin production. When serotonin production is restored, your cravings will disappear, making it possible to overcome habits and addictions that weaken and exhaust the adrenal glands.

When you want to get off SSRIs, I encourage you *not* to go cold turkey. Make sure you are working with your doctor and perhaps a natural health care practitioner such as a naturopath, chiropractor, herbalist, nutritionist, or acupuncturist. Begin improving your diet and lifestyle by following the Ten Simple Solutions.

When you are consumed with a myriad of details and demands, it is easy to slide into habits that deplete your adrenal reserve. As the adrenal reserve diminishes, turning to stimulants is common. When stimulants no longer make you feel better, drugs are often thought of as the solution. Sugar, stimulants, and drugs are highly addicting because they make burned-out people feel better temporarily. But they are wolves in sheep's clothing. After the good feelings pass, these wolves will devour what is left of your adrenal reserve and your health.

By following the Ten Simple Solutions, you can feel better enough to wean yourself from sugar, stimulants, and drugs.

Many learned behaviors start in childhood, going back to Mom's cookies. The first foods we eat end up producing certain comforting sensations and responses—and these foods are often the hardest habits to kick. With any addiction—whether it is sugar, heroin, or nicotine—there will be a withdrawal period when you quit. To avoid the physical and emotional pain of going cold turkey, give your body the precursors to make serotonin. Whether you are giving up coffee, cigarettes, SSRIs, cocaine, or Mom's chocolate chip cookies, giving your body the necessary building blocks in the form of supplements and real, whole foods will make this process easier.

Quitting Addictions and Getting off Antidepressants

Formula for Defeating Sugar Cravings

Take an herbal formula that contains:

- 450 milligrams St. John's wort bud

If you cannot take St. John's wort, you can substitute 500 milligrams L-tryptophan or 100 milligrams 5HTP twice a day. You can ask your doctor for a prescription for L-tryptophan. 5HTP is available in health food stores. *This formula is not intended for people who are currently taking SSRIs or MAO inhibitors.*

Replenishing Formulas to Boost Serotonin to Aid in Defeating Sugar Cravings and in Quitting Addictions

To avoid the physical and emotional pain of going cold turkey when you quit addictions, give your body the necessary building blocks to make serotonin. *The following formula is not intended for people who are currently taking SSRIs or MAO inhibitors.*

One-half hour before breakfast, lunch, and dinner and before bedtime take an herbal formula that contains:

450 milligrams St. John's wort

and an herbal decoction of sour jujube seed, California poppy whole plant, red sage root, hawthorn berry, St. John's wort

If this formula does not ease your cravings, or if you cannot take St. John's wort, you may try the following formulas. This formula is not intended for people who are currently taking SSRIs or MAO inhibitors.

On a relatively empty stomach, with something sweet such as one-quarter apple and a few almonds to balance the sugar, take 500 milligrams L-tryptophan—by prescription only. If you do not see any improvement within two weeks, increase to 1,000 milligrams.

Also add: 25 milligrams vitamin B6

and 100 milligrams magnesium

or

On a relatively empty stomach, with something sweet such as one-quarter apple and a bite of cheese to balance the sugar, take 100 milligrams of 5-HTP. If you do not see any improvement within two weeks, increase to 1,000 milligrams.

Also add: 25 milligrams vitamin B6

and 100 milligrams magnesium

You may take this formula to your health food store and research the products that match this formula as closely as possible. You will find product-ordering information on page 355. You can ask your doctor for a prescription for L-tryptophan. 5-HTP, vitamin B6, and magnesium are available in health food stores.

Other factors that will help raise
serotonin production

___ Eat protein at every meal or snack. The power drink recipes in chapter 15 beginning on page 334 will help.

___ Practice deep breathing, which nourishes and recharges your system while inducing relaxation and clarity. Indulge in slow, deep breathing all day long, especially before meals.

___ Provide your body with the vitamins, minerals, and other nutrients you need to repair and to loosen the stranglehold of your addiction. Your personal program can be found in chapter 9.

___ Do what you can to eliminate white flour and sugar.

___ Avoid processed, junk, and fake foods and/or chemicals.

___ Drink organic green tea, which has half the caffeine of coffee, is filled with antioxidants, and does not contain pesticides.

___ Drink a detox tea.

___ Practice positive thinking to change your psychogene.

___ Have some fun every day.

___ Engage in moderate exercise that you find fun and that clears your mind.

___ Be in sunshine every day, if possible.

___ Pray and listen to inspiring music.

Simple Solution 5: Let Go of Your Favorite Poison
Tailored to your stage of burnout

Driven and Dragging

___ You are on top of the world now. Why trade that good feel for cravings, mood swings, and depression? If you stop eating sugar now, you can avoid the blood sugar roller coaster that will deplete your adrenal reserve, break down muscle mass, and decrease your metabolism.

___ Eating regular balanced meals of real, whole foods will pre-

vent you from developing cravings and ruining your great
metabolism.

___ Caffeine is an insidious part of our culture. You do not have
to conform to this unhealthy habit. If you have a caffeine
habit, you can wean gently off by following the serotonin-
boosting guidelines on page 206–208, and by taking the recommended supplements for your stage of burnout.

___ If you are a smoker, and you quit smoking now, you will
thank yourself later. Make it easier to kick the nicotine habit
with the help of the serotonin-boosting formulas on pages
206–208, and take the recommended supplements for your
stage of burnout.

Losing It and Hitting the Wall

___ Your sugar habit has resulted in cravings and mood swings.
You have less muscle mass and your metabolism is notice-
ably slower than it used to be. You feel a little depressed. If
you stop eating now, you can avoid further adrenal damage
from the blood sugar roller coaster.

___ It is more important than ever to begin eating regular balanced meals of real, whole foods to end your hunger and
cravings for sweets.

___ Have you noticed that caffeine does not really do the trick
any more? Gently wean off caffeine with the help of the
serotonin-boosting guidelines on pages 206–208, and take
the recommended supplements for your stage of burnout.

___ If you smoke, your dependence on cigarettes is a ball and
chain you hate. You can make it easier to kick nicotine with
the help of the serotonin-boosting guidelines on pages
206–208, and take the recommended supplements for your
stage of burnout.

___ Stop using herbal stimulants with the help of the serotonin-
boosting guidelines on pages 206–208, and take the recommended supplements for your stage of burnout.

___ Work with your doctor and perhaps a natural health care practitioner such as a naturopath, chiropractor, or acupuncturist to quit tranquilizers and antidepressants. Make the transition easier by following the serotonin-boosting guidelines on pages 206–208, and take the recommended supplements for your stage of burnout.

___ If you have started taking SSRIs, sooner or later you are going to suffer from SSRIs burnout. Why wait? Wean from SSRIs by working with your doctor and perhaps a natural health care practitioner such as a naturopath, chiropractor, herbalist, nutritionist, or acupuncturist. Follow the serotonin-boosting guidelines on pages 206–208, and the recommended supplements for your stage of burnout.

Burned Out

___ Eating sugar is deadly at this stage. Cravings, mood swings, and depression can all end. Stop eating sugar to end the blood sugar roller coaster that has depleted your adrenal reserve, broken down muscle mass, and decreased your metabolism.

___ Eating regular balanced meals of real, whole foods is critical to end your hunger and cravings for sweets and to restore adrenal function.

___ Caffeine will keep you in a holding pattern of adrenal burnout. You do not need caffeine—or even decaffeinated coffee at this point. Wean off caffeine gently with the help of the serotonin-boosting guidelines on pages 206–208, and by taking the recommended supplements for your stage of burnout.

___ Kick the nicotine habit now to save your life. You can do it with the help of the serotonin-boosting guidelines on pages 206–208, and by taking the recommended supplements for your stage of burnout.

___ Using herbal stimulants will continue to deplete your already ravaged adrenal glands. Avoid them or quit using them with the help of the serotonin-boosting guidelines on pages 206–208, and by taking the recommended supplements for your stage of burnout.

___ Tranquilizers and antidepressants will not heal you, but you may need them to get through this stage. When you are ready, you can wean off these substances with the help of your doctor and perhaps a natural health care practitioner such as a naturopath, chiropractor, or acupuncturist. Use the serotonin-boosting guidelines on pages 206–208, and take the recommended supplements for your stage of burnout.

___ Likewise, SSRIs will not be in your life forever, but you may need this life raft now. When you are ready, you can wean from SSRIs by working with your doctor and perhaps a natural health care practitioner such as a naturopath, chiropractor, herbalist, nutritionist, or acupuncturist. Follow the serotonin-boosting guidelines on pages 206–208, and take the recommended supplements for your stage of burnout.

Simple Solution 6
Supplement a Tired Food Chain

*Our depleted food sources must
be augmented with vitamins,
minerals, and other nutrients*

Shortcuts to Simple Solution 6

• To replace what is missing in our depleted food
sources, take a daily vitamin/mineral supplement.

• Take herbs, therapeutic nutrients, amino acids,
and hormones appropriate for your stage
of adrenal burnout.

Vitamins and minerals are the catalysts of cellular
function. Without adequate vitamins and minerals your cellular function will falter and fail. This leads to diminished vitality and premature degeneration—or aging. Vitamins and minerals are the humus from which your body creates life and are an essential part of restoring adrenal function. Since the human body cannot

make vitamins and minerals, they have to be obtained from an external source—which in the past was food. However, farmlands have been overcultivated and depleted of nutrients, so the majority of the food in our food chain contains barely half of the vitamins and minerals it contained fifty years ago. Unfortunately, there is not yet enough organic farming on rejuvenated farmland for the escalating demands of our society. And unless you have a garden in your backyard, even organic foods are not perfect. For example, by the time a cabbage is picked, shipped, and stocked on the grocery shelf seventy-two hours later, it has lost most of its vitamin C.

More than at any time in history, we have placed frightening demands on our bodies by eating refined and adulterated foods that are so devoid of nutrients that even bugs cannot live on them. We ingest stimulants and drugs, and we are exposed to gamma rays from air travel X-rays and ionizing radiation from computers and other appliances, and irradiated foods. We are exposed to pesticides and herbicides, heavy metals, PCBs, DDT, and other poisons. These poisons damage cellular function, which will ultimately damage metabolism. In addition, as we age, we do not absorb nutrients as well. All of these challenges require an extra therapeutic intake of vitamins and minerals for cellular function and rebuilding as well as detoxification. Medical literature is replete with studies that demonstrate that we really do make a difference in our vitality, recovery, and regeneration when we eat well and take good supplements.

Of course it would be better if we obtained nutrients in their native form in foods. Since we have to get our nutrients somewhere, vitamin and mineral supplements have evolved to fill this role. On the other hand, supplements are meant to augment a diet of whole, real foods. Vitamin and mineral supplements *fill in* what is missing in your diet and is required by your body. They *cannot substitute for good nutrition.* On a balanced diet of real, whole foods, you can repair and replenish your adrenals. On a diet of refined foods, even though you may take vitamin and mineral supplements, it is only a matter of time before all the empty foods leave you so malnourished that you are weakened and wounded.

Just as I advise people to eat a variety of foods, we need to take adequate amounts of a variety of vitamins and minerals. I prescribe amounts of vitamins and minerals that are above the Food and Drug Administration's (FDA) recommended daily allowance (RDA) for a number of reasons. When the RDAs were first created in the 1940s, healthy medical students were evaluated to determine the average nutritional needs of average people. This was before the decline in the quality of farming and the systematic refining of foods—when food was still loaded with nutrients. Nowadays our food does not contain the same nutritional density as it did in the 1940s, and at the same time we have increased demands on our bodies. Lately, health practitioners like myself are using our own clinical experience to create upgraded recommended optimal vitamin and mineral allowances.

Your body is smart enough to pick out the nutrients it needs from food, when available, and it is smart enough to pick and choose the nutrients it needs from the vitamin/mineral supplements you take. We thrive when our bodies are given the opportunity to choose from *abundance*. You may have heard people say that if you take vitamins you have expensive urine because the body eliminates what it does not immediately need. The good news is that when you take adequate amounts of vitamins and minerals, you may have expensive urine, but you also have a nutrient-rich bloodstream that is bathing your cells with nutrients for optimal repair and regeneration.

Vitamins A and D are oil-soluble vitamins that concentrate in the liver and become toxic if taken in excess. I do not recommend these vitamins outside of the multiple vitamin/mineral supplement that contains adequate yet safe levels of each.

Because vitamins and minerals work synergistically in the metabolic and enzymatic systems in our bodies, we need to take vitamins and minerals in certain combinations. The proper combination can be found in a good-quality multiple vitamin/mineral supplement. Although we can use a particular vitamin or mineral therapeutically in response to a symptomatic need, by doing so we often create an increased need for other vitamins and minerals. That is why I am convinced that it is best to take the right combinations in a multiple first—as the cornerstone of good nutrition. When conditions persist that indicate specific nutrient deficiencies, therapeutic amounts of individual vitamins and minerals and all the other healing supplements can be added to accelerate repair.

Since vitamin/mineral supplements fill in what is missing in our food, they are *always* best absorbed when taken with food, when your digestive juices are flowing. But even with food, if you were to take a handful of vitamin and mineral pills all at once the absorptive surfaces of your intestines would be overwhelmed. For that reason I recommend a multiple vitamin/mineral supplement that contains smaller amounts of each vitamin and mineral in every pill to be taken with food two to six times a day depending on your stage of adrenal burnout. By taking these capsules throughout the day, your body has a better chance of absorbing and utilizing these smaller amounts and you will waste less in expensive urine. Amounts of the vitamins and minerals I recommend in a multiple can be found starting on page 228. Product-ordering information can be found on page 355.

You may be familiar with many of these vitamins and minerals, but let's take a look at a few of them in relation to adrenal burnout.

Vitamins

VITAMIN A: A powerful antioxidant; improves and balances immunity.

BIOTIN: Essential for the activity of many enzyme systems.

CHOLINE: A memory nutrient.

INOSITOL: An antidepressant and a sugar specific for muscles.

VITAMIN C (ASCORBIC ACID): A building block for adrenal steroid biosynthesis. Vitamin C is depleted from the adrenal cortex when cortisol is being secreted.

CITRUS BIOFLAVONOID COMPLEX: Bioflavonoids are phytonutrients that stablize cell membranes, balance hormones, and are antiinflammatory.

VITAMIN D: Needed for calcium and phosphorus absorption.

VITAMIN E: An amazing antioxidant, vitamin E is a fat-soluble vitamin that improves circulation, tissue repair, healing, fibrocystic conditions, and PMS.

PARA-AMINOBENZOIC ACID (PABA): Aids hormone metabolism.

VITAMIN B COMPLEXES: B vitamins are useful in nearly every aspect of our energy and repair systems, including the production and the effect of hormones, antibiotics, and neurotransmitters. For adrenal burnout I recommend equal amounts vitamin B1, B2, B3, and B6. B5 needs to be taken in higher amounts, B12 in smaller amounts. Recommendations are included in the vitamin/mineral lists.

VITAMIN B1 (THIAMIN): Essential to carbohydrate metabolism and a healthy nervous system; is depleted rapidly by alcohol, which can result in memory loss.

VITAMIN B2 (RIBOFLAVIN): Protects skin, mouth, eyes, eyelids, and mucous membranes; essential to protein and energy metabolism; effectively diminishes migraines in some people.

VITAMIN B3 (NIACIN): This vitamin is a cofactor of steroid biosynthesis; is critical for healthy liver function; is a vasodilator (relaxes blood vessels), improves circulation and lowers cholesterol. Doses over 25 milligrams may cause a hot flash from the stimulation of the rapid relaxation of blood cells as they are flushing toxins and wastes out. It is not dangerous, but some people do not like this sensation.

VITAMIN B5 (PANTOTHENIC ACID): Stimulates the energy-making systems in the body and is used in the biosynthesis of adrenaline and cortisol. A dose of vitamin B5 in addition to a multiple vitamin, along with better eating habits, can be all it takes to provide what your body needs to recover from adrenal burnout in the early stages of burnout.

VITAMIN B6 (PYRIDOXINE): Helps regulate the central nervous system and helps metabolize proteins and hormones. A natural diuretic and critical for healthy hormonal metabolism and neurotransmitters.

FOLIC ACID OR FOLATE: Used in the biosynthesis of adrenaline and cortisol, required for normal blood cell formation, growth, and reproduction and for many important chemical reactions in cells.

VITAMIN B12 (COBALAMIN): Necessary to the formation of all blood cells and maintaining healthy nerves and heart. It protects some genes from genetic mutation.

Minerals

Minerals, like vitamins, are catalysts for many systems, especially the energy-producing endocrine glands such as thyroid and adrenal.

CALCIUM: A natural calming agent that is depleted by stress and must be replenished. When calcium is diminished, you feel more agitated. Many women are eating antacids to get their calcium, but antacids neutralize the very acid that is required to absorb calcium under any circumstances. Furthermore, the calcium carbonate found in antacids is the very hardest type of calcium to absorb.

CHROMIUM: Helps insulin to function as a blood sugar normalizer. Daily use of 200 to 400 micrograms is considered below any potential toxicity.

COPPER AND ZINC: These minerals are depleted by stress and must be replenished. They are best taken together; otherwise one could cause a depletion of the other. They are best in a ratio of zinc 20 milligrams to copper 2 milligrams.

IODINE: Important for thyroid metabolism.

IRON: Critical for red blood cells to carry oxygen to your cells.

MAGNESIUM: Calming to the nervous system, it is involved in over one hundred metabolic enzyme reactions in the body. It is an important cofactor in the production of neurotransmitters and helps alleviate muscle spasms, fibromyalgia, allergies, constipation, and PMS. I use oral magnesium in my practice to relieve the muscle spasms in the intestinal tract that cause constipation. When the sympathetic nervous system is dominant, the intestinal tract tightens and shuts down. Magnesium relaxes the intestinal grip so that digestion can take place.

MANGANESE: Is involved in the health of connective tissues such as ligaments, tendons, and bones and is the catalyst for numerous enzymatic reactions.

POTASSIUM: This mineral is depleted by stress and must be replenished. Potassium deficiencies can cause fatal heartbeat irregularities and/or cramps, spasms, and twitches anywhere in the body. Potassium helps keep our systems alkaline enough during the day and activates the alkaline tide of Rest, Repair, and Rejuvenation at night.

SELENIUM: A well-recognized antioxidant that is considered important to prevent cancer.

VANADIUM (VANADYL SULFATE): Helps normalize and maintain insulin receptor functions. Without vandadyl sulfate, you are more likely to have insulin resistance and type II diabetes.

Antioxidants

A free radical is a molecule with at least one unpaired electron. Free radicals are formed during normal metabolic processes as energy is produced in the cells. They are also produced by cigarette smoke, exhaust, insecticides, and other poisons. Even seemingly benign household products such as hairspray and detergents generate free radicals.

Free radicals are further generated when normal molecules meet up with free radical molecules that are missing electrons. Since electrons must be paired, these once-peaceful molecules become like angry gang members looking to cause trouble everywhere. Free radicals race around your body trying to pair with other electrons by stealing electrons from other molecules, which creates oxidation. Oxidation is defined as any reaction involving a loss of electrons. Excess oxidation accelerates aging and damages the energy factories in cells. This can lead to premature aging, degenerative disease, and abnormal weight gain. The consumption of unhealthy oils (explained in chapter 4) also contributes to excess oxidation in the body.

An antioxidant is a substance that prevents or slows oxidation. Studies show that antioxidants in the body, such as vitamins E and C and beta-carotene—a vitamin A precursor—can prevent cell damage and other changes caused by oxidation. Antioxidants scavenge the free radicals that cause oxidation. All the antioxidants you need for good health are contained in the basic multiple vitamin/mineral formula.

ALPHA-CAROTENE, CRYPTOXANTHIN, LUTEIN, AND ZEAXANTHIN: are all wonderful antioxidants that are part of the multiple vitamin/mineral supplement.

Sodium

Although sodium is not included in a multiple vitamin/mineral supplement, it is an essential mineral for restoring adrenal function. Historically, wars were fought over salt. Although current research has demonstrated that only ten percent of people suffering from hypertension need to restrict salt intake, many people are still operating under the old assumption that salt should be severely restricted.

Our bodies contain fluids such as blood plasma and lymphatic fluids that closely resemble the electrical balance and chemical composition of ocean water. We need a little salt to replace the salt that is lost through daily sweating and urinating. In stressful times our adrenals need sodium to function properly. The later the stage of adrenal exhaustion, the more likely you are to need salt. And the lower your blood pressure, which is another sign of adrenal exhaustion, the more salt you need. Anyone under stress should not be on a no-salt diet, unless advised otherwise by his or her doctor. If you crave salt, there may be a good reason. Of course, there is also a difference between irrational cravings and cravings for something your body needs—so there is a common-sense limit to the amount of salt you can safely use.

Processed foods contain an overabundance of table salt. This salt should be used only for melting snow and other industrial uses, not for human consumption. Regular table salt has had most of the trace minerals removed during the refining process; they are sold to the chemical industry or to pharmaceutical companies to make dietary supplements. Regular table salt contains sodium chloride, with little or no minerals and with sugar as filler, and it may even contain aluminum.

Ocean salt contains all of the precious minerals your body's systems require. The best salt is Celtic Sea salt, which is filled with trace minerals as well as sodium and potassium salts. Celtic Sea salt is obtained from the evaporation of the ocean's water in Brittany, near the Celtic Sea, in the northwest of France. Kosher salts are not usually true sea salt.

This information is not meant to contradict the advice of your doctor. If you have been put on a low-sodium diet, consult with your doctor before making any adjustments in your sodium intake.

Additional Supplements

Herbs, therapeutic nutrients, amino acids, and hormones are also important for adrenal rejuvenation. It is important that you do not overdo any of these types of supplements. I encourage giving the body adequate amounts of vitamins and minerals; unfortunately, in our culture people tend to the extreme. If someone takes one ginseng capsule and finds that they feel better, too often they think ten will be better. Not true. The goal with these nutrients is to give your body an amount as close as possible to what it needs. Furthermore, the needs for each stage of adrenal burnout differ. For example, if you are in the Driven stage, you do not need the herbs I have listed here. Herbs might act as stimulants and would be as destructive as using any other stimulant. If you do not need herbs and take them for their stimulant effect, they can cause the feelings of a panic attack. In later stages herbs can help restore adrenal function, but they are not to be taken in place of all of the other important steps. You cannot keep driving your adrenals and take supplements and expect repair to happen. Herbs, therapeutic nutrients, amino acids, glandulars, and hormones should be used in addition to the other steps to support your system while the healing processes are taking place.

Herbs

ALOE LEAF EXTRACT: Valued for its immune-enhancing and mucous membrane–healing capabilities.

ASHWAGANDA: Considered by many to be the Ayurvedic equivalent of ginseng; an adaptagenic herb that improves adrenal function. A tonic for mental energy and a general system tonic.

HOLY BASIL: An adaptogenic herb; nourishes and supports adrenal function. Lowers excess cortisol and protects your adrenal reserve and helps spare your adrenals from being damaged by the demands placed on them through chronic stress. Also helps balance blood sugar.

KAVA KAVA: A South Pacific herb known for its calming effects. When standardized extracts of the kavalactones are used—100 to 300 milligrams, between one and four times a day as needed—there is no known toxicity. Used in the massive doses common among the South Sea islanders, it can be hallucinogenic and can cause extreme lethargy, ambivalence, lack of ambition, and even reptilian-like scales.

LICORICE ROOT: An adaptogenic (balancing) herb that improves adrenal function. Licorice root contains glycyrrhizic (*gli sear rye zik*) acid, which prolongs the availability of the cortisol your body has made so that your body and brain do not perceive as much of a constant increased demand. Again, in our culture people think that if a little is good then a lot has to be better, and people have been known to take too much licorice root. There is a small group of people in whom licorice root raises blood pressure and alters potassium levels. So even though licorice root is extremely effective in adrenal support, if you take significant amounts, you need to be aware that it can raise blood pressure. You are advised to have your blood pressure checked regularly and your potassium levels checked occasionally to make sure that they stay within normal ranges. However, deglycyrrhinated licorice root does not affect blood pressure, potassium levels, or adrenal function. People who have low blood pressure because their adrenals are weak can find that licorice root will restore adrenal function, which will result in normalizing their blood pressure.

MARSHMALLOW ROOT: This herb is soothing and coating and therefore protective of the gastrointestinal tract.

ROYAL MACCA: I consider royal macca to be the Peruvian equivalent of ginseng. An adaptagenic herb, it improves adrenal function and has many nourishing adrenal support and balancing qualities. It improves virility, energy, and stamina and balances hormones.

SIBERIAN GINSENG: An adaptogenic herb that has been used for approximately four thousand years and is well researched and widely respected. It supports the body during times of stress. It was used in the past by Russian athletes and emperors for its ability to increase optimal mental and physical performance. It nourishes the adrenals and is a general system tonic. For adrenal support it is considered superior to American and Korean ginseng.

SILYMARIN (MILK THISTLE SEED), BUPLERUM, DANDELION ROOT, BEET LEAVES, BURDOCK, GOLDENSEAL: These herbs are commonly used liver-nourishing herbs; they repair, support, and protect liver function. Most people who are suffering from adrenal burnout have consumed substances that have exhausted or damaged their liver.

ST. JOHN'S WORT: Has been used in Europe for decades to treat depressive disorders. It is thought that St. John's wort increases serotonin levels and lowers cortisol levels.

VALERIANA, PASSAFLORA, AND HOPS: These herbs have been used for hundreds of years for their calming effects. I use combinations of these herbs for relaxation, anxiety, and sleep.

Therapeutic Nutrients

COLOSTRUM: This nutrient is a distillate of cow milk. When a mammal gives birth, before the onset of true lactation, a thin, yellowish substance is secreted called colostrum. It contains a great quantity of antibodies—"information" proteins that provide direction to the immune system, and lymphocytes, which are the main means of providing the body with immune capability.

PHOSPHATIDYLSERINE (FOS FOE TITLE SER EENE): When incorporated into the cell membrane, phosphatidylserine improves and maintains brain function. Phosphatidylserine is a brain nutrient that helps rebalance pituitary/adrenal communication and nourishes and supports your adrenals while you rest. It influences your brain to diminish the production of the adrenal releasing factor, so that your adrenals do not get the message to inappropriately release cortisol and DHEA. For those who suffer from insomnia because their adrenals are turning on inappropriately at night, phosphatidylserine can help to diminish this inappropriate activation of your adrencls.

QUERCETIN: An antioxidant bioflavonoid—a phytonutrient—that quells allergy reactions.

Amino Acids

There are twenty amino acids that are important for human metabolism. Ten can be produced within the body and are referred to as nonessential. The other ten, which are required for life but not made in the body, are referred to as essential amino acids. These must be obtained by eating protein or by taking supplements. Amino acids are building blocks of protein structures in the body such as hair, nails, muscle, and bone. To make these structures, for any amino acid to be absorbed into your brain and not with the rest of your food, it must be taken on a relatively empty stomach. Amino acids are best taken with a little bit of something sweet such as ¼ cup fruit juice with a small amount of protein to balance the sugar so that insulin will assist absorption directly into the brain.

5H-GAMMA AMINOBUTYRIC ACID (5-H GABA) AND GAMMA AMINO-
BUTYRIC ACID (GABA) (GAMMA AMEENO BYEW TEAR IC ACID):
Both increase the amount of calming neurotransmitters in your
brain. In fact, they produce the same calming effect as Valium and
are used to alleviate panic attacks. The difference between 5-H GABA
and GABA and Valium is that drugs such as Valium mimic our calming neurotransmitters while 5-H GABA and GABA nourish and replenish these neurotransmitters. For this reason 5-H GABA and
GABA are nonaddictive. From the stages Dragging through Burned
Out your adrenals are exhausted, and any further demand will only
further fatigue and deplete them. During this hyperstimulation
phase of adrenal burnout, you will begin to feel more agitated. 5-H
GABA and GABA can be effective in calming this anxiety. 5-H GABA
is a more usable form than GABA, which is why you need a smaller
dose. Both are equally effective.

GLUTAMINE: An amazing amino acid that helps balance blood sugar
and liver function and increases the level of critical antioxidants.
When taken at night, glutamine helps alkalinize your body and increases level of human growth hormone—a hormone that helps balance all the other systems in our body and is the most potent
longevity hormone known. The cells that line our intestinal tract
need glutamine, and when it is present in proper amounts it speeds
up the healing of intestinal problems.

GLYCINE: Best known for diminishing sugar and alcohol cravings.

LYSINE: An antiviral.

L-TRYPTOPHAN: The precursor to serotonin and melatonin; obtained
by prescription only. (At one time, L-tryptophan was the leading
solution for sleep disturbances. In the late 1980s, a contaminated
batch of L-tryptophan caused muscular problems and one death.
The source of the problem turned out to be a toxic substance that
had slipped into the manufacturer's product, not L-tryptophan. Nonetheless, L-tryptophan was taken off the market.) L-tryptophan is a
precursor to the calming neurotransmitters serotonin and mela-

tonin; it can calm sleep disturbances and help lift depression. It is usually taken at nighttime for its calming effect, but it can be taken throughout the day for its antidepressant effect. And if someone is very agitated, it can be taken all day. It may take up to three weeks to notice the calming effects, so please be patient. *Note: Do not take L-tryptophan if you are taking SSRIs such as Prozac or Zoloft.*

5-HYDROXY TRYPTOPHAN (5-HTP): A more usable form of L-tryptophan; can be obtained over the counter. 5-HTP is considered to be five times more potent than L-tryptophan—so you do not need to take as much. *Note: Do not take 5-HTP if you are taking SSRIs such as Prozac or Zoloft.*

TYROSINE: A precursor to norepinephrine, epinephrine (adrenaline), dopamine, and thyroid hormone, which are the energy-providing hormones of the body. *Note: Do not take tyrosine if you are taking MAO inhibitors. The three main MAO inhibitors currently used in the United States are Nardil, Reserpine, and Parnate.*

Hormones

Natural hormones made from plants are an exact match of human hormones. They are safe only when taken in physiologic doses so that you maintain normal blood or saliva levels. In other words, hormones are only safe when taken to replace the amount you cannot produce in your body. Hormone imbalances can cause serious health problems. If you take hormones, it is wise to be monitored by a health care practitioner who is knowledgeable in natural hormone replacement therapy.

DIHYDROEPIANDROSTERONE (DI HYDRO EPI AN DROSS TERONE) (DHEA): This is the balancing hormone to cortisol. DHEA improves immunity, stimulates fat burning, improves energy, and is reported to improve longevity, treat chronic fatigue, and suppress autoimmune diseases. Many people who are extremely exhausted are not making enough DHEA. In several instances I have seen appropriate replacement doses of DHEA dramatically improve chronic fatigue.

An average woman secretes 10 to 20 milligrams of DHEA a day, and an average man secretes 15 to 30 milligrams of DHEA a day. We are fairly new at exploring and understanding DHEA. When it comes to taking any hormone that has not been extensively studied and clinically tested over long periods of time, it is best to not risk the unknown. Use DHEA in physiologic amounts: this means an amount that would be normal for your body to produce on its own. Pharmacological doses—above what a human body would normally make on its own—could have unknown side effects that may not show up for a decade or two.

DHEA levels can be checked through saliva tests. A normal dose of DHEA for a woman is between 5 and 20 milligrams per day, depending on her stage of burnout and how well she absorbs it. A normal dose for a man is between 10 and 50 milligrams per day, depending on how well he absorbs it and his stage of burnout. It is important to note that in some people DHEA causes acne, hair loss on your head, and hair growth on your face—or hair in "all the wrong places."

HUMAN GROWTH HORMONE (hGH): This hormone helps balance all the other systems in the body and is the most potent longevity hormone known. The natural decline of human growth hormone often parallels aging and burnout. The replacement of hGH secretion has been observed to regenerate and repair most systems, including the adrenals.

Some people cannot wind down at night to get to sleep; they do not have enough alkaline reserve in their systems to slide into the nighttime parasympathetic repair biochemistry. HGH increases melatonin and improves sleep. Many people who cannot relax at night find they sleep better when they take homeopathic human growth hormone. I have patients who have had spectacular reversals of insomnia by using hGH.

MELATONIN: The pineal gland is a pea-sized organ situated in the brain that registers day and night by sensing light and dark and regulates the body's circadian rhythm—a daily rhythmic activity cycle, based on twenty-four-hour intervals. The pineal gland produces a hormone called melatonin in periods of darkness, which makes you feel sleepy and aids in turning on the nighttime Rest, Repair, and Rejuvenation processes. The brain's ability to make the hormone melatonin decreases with age. So if you are suffering from insomnia, melatonin is a good first step. While melatonin has been tested and found to be extremely safe in a low dose, there are those who have a paradoxical reaction, wherein melatonin causes them to feel energized or to have nightmares. This is not life threatening but is obviously not the goal, and if it happens you should try the other formulas recommended throughout this book.

Chinese Herbs

Chinese medicine is a three-thousand-year-old healing art that uses herbs instead of drugs. Chinese herbology is respected as one of the most sophisticated medical modalities in the world.

There are over four hundred commonly used herbs in Chinese medicine. Herbal formulas contain specific combinations of roots, seeds, grains, flowers, berries, fruit peel, bark, leaves, stems, kernels, wood, shells, nuts, minerals, pollen, resin, seaweed, clay, fossilized bones, and occasionally animal proteins. Each herb in a formula has multiple active ingredients that result in various effects on the body. When combined, these herbs can produce, potentially, a nearly infinite number of interactions.

Chinese herbs are often effective in treating chronic conditions that defy traditional Western medicine.

Putting it all together

Each person has unique nutrient requirements created by their level of stress and personal genetic factors. We do not yet have dependable and trustworthy testing to determine exact individual supplement needs. Your body is the best laboratory. Pay attention. Start on supplements slowly. *Do not begin to take all of the supplements all at once. Do not combine supplements that are meant to be taken separately.* Begin with one or two multiple vitamin/mineral capsules that are similar to the formula I describe on page 228. The following day, add one or two more and continue increasing until you reach the recommended dose for your stage. Then you may begin to add super green foods. Next, I encourage you to increase vitamin B5. I prefer the rest of the supplements to be added slowly. For each stage, I have laid out an easy-to-follow daily plan for you to integrate these supplements into your daily routine.

Please make changes in your body gradually. Overloading your body with nutrients that it cannot possibly absorb or utilize—and that might even be dangerous when taken in extreme amounts—is counterproductive and really will not benefit you in the short or long run. If you have negative reactions to any nutritional supplement, immediately discontinue the apparent cause, make a note, and try again at a later day.

Your tailored supplement program includes formulas that I consider optimal. It is important in your healing process for you to take the best quality supplements. The criteria for supplements are: 1) truth in labeling, 2) the most absorbable form of each nutrient, and 3) the least amount of fillers and binders. Not all supplements companies create quality products. Unless you are an expert, it is impossible to know which products are inferior and which are superior. For that reason, I have listed the names of several reputable companies on page 355.

Daily Vitamins

A complete list follows of the vitamins and minerals I recommend you look for in a daily supplement. *This is not a formula for pregnancy.*

Daily vitamin and mineral supplement
(These amounts are the total of six pills.)

vitamin A: 5,000 IU
beta-carotene: 15,000 IU
vitamin E: 400 IU—it should
   be D-alpha, which is natural, not DL-alpha, which is
   synthetic
vitamin D (calciferol): 20 IU
vitamin C: 1,200 milligrams

B3 (niacinamide, niacin): 120
   milligrams
hydrochloric acid: 325
   milligrams
choline (bitartrate): 200
   milligrams
inositol: 188 milligrams
vitamin B5: 500 milligrams
citrus bioflavonoid complex:
   100 milligrams
PABA: 50 milligrams
vitamin B6: 40 milligrams
vitamin B2: 34 milligrams
vitamin B1: 30 milligrams
folic acid: 800 micrograms
biotin: 300 micrograms
vitamin B12: 200 micrograms
calcium (citrate): 500
   milligrams
magnesium (glycinate
   citrate): 250 milligrams—
   decrease amount if you
   experience loose bowels
potassium (aspartate): 99
   milligrams

iron (glycinate): 10
   milligrams
zinc (aspartate): 20
   milligrams
manganese (aspartate): 1
   milligram
copper (lysinate): 2
   milligrams
chromium (dinicotinate
   glycinate): 200 micrograms
selenium (aspartate): 200
   micrograms
iodine (potassium iodide):
   150 micrograms
molybdenum (aspartate):
   100 micrograms
vanadium (vanadyl sulfate):
   39 micrograms
quercetin: 25 milligrams
alpha-carotene: 132
   micrograms
cryptoxanthin: 32
   micrograms
zeaxanthin: 28 micrograms
lutein: 20 micrograms

Super green food

Look for super green food formulas that contain a blend of freeze-dried, antioxidant-rich mixed vegetable powders such as carrot, tomato, and broccoli; anti-aging herbs such as turmeric, green tea, and Siberian ginseng; freeze-dried cereal grasses such as barley and wheat; liver-supporting herbs such as milk thistle seed, ginko biloba,

pycnogenol (an antioxidant from grape seed), as well as freeze-dried
sea vegetables such as spirulina and chlorella. See page 355 for product recommendations.

Formulas That May Be Added If You Are in the Dragging Through Burned Out Stages

Integrate any of the following formulas slowly. Remember, the body
will be a little sensitive at any stage of adrenal burnout, so make sure
you listen carefully to its signals.

DHEA

If you are in Hitting the Wall or Burned Out, this is a good time to
start DHEA. You can find DHEA at your health food store.

WOMEN: 1 milligram DHEA. If you do not see any improvement after
one week, increase 1 milligram per week up to 15 milligrams.

MEN: 5 milligrams DHEA. If you do not see any improvement after
one week, increase 1 to 2 milligrams each week up to 25 milligrams.

Human Growth Hormone (hGH)

Human Growth Hormone (hGH) helps balance all the other systems
in the body and is the most potent longevity hormone known. The
natural decline of human growth hormone often parallels aging and
burnout. The replacement of hGH secretion has been observed to
regenerate and repair most systems, including the adrenals. If you are
in Losing It, Hitting the Wall, or Burned Out stage, this is a good time
to start hGH. You can obtain homeopathic hGH from your health
care practitioner.

Fatigue formula

    300 milligrams of licorice root
    50 milligrams ashwaganda

An herbal decoction containing rehmannia root, schizandra fruit, jujube fruit, don quai root, asparagus root, ophiopogon root, scrophularia root, codonopsis root, saliva root, poria sclerotium, polygala root, and platycodon root

Simple Solution 6: Supplement a Tired Food Chain Tailored to your stage of adrenal burnout

Driven

___ You cannot take supplements and continue your behavior with impunity. You need basic supplements to make up for the vitamin and mineral deficiencies in food.

___ Take the properly formulated daily vitamin/mineral supplement to supply your body with abundant nutrients.

___ Adding a power drink made with super green food is a good insurance policy.

Driven	Breakfast	Dinner
Day 1-3	Multi-Vit/Min 2 Green Food caps.	Multi-Vit/Min 2 Green Food caps.
Day 4 onward	Multi-Vit/Min 2 Green Food caps.	Multi-Vit/Min 2 Green Food caps.

Dragging

___ Taking the properly formulated daily vitamin/mineral supplement to supply your body with abundant nutrients will help stave off further adrenal fatigue.

___ Take the amino acids and herbs that are appropriate for your stage of adrenal burnout.

___ Power drinks made with green food will help nourish your adrenal glands.

Dragging	Pre-breakfast	Breakfast	Lunch	By 3:30 p.m.	Dinner
Day 1-3		Multi-Vit/Min 2 Green Food caps.			
Day 4-6		Multi-Vit/Min 2 Green Food caps.			Multi-Vit/Min 2 Green Food caps.
Day 7-9		Multi-Vit/Min 2 Green Food caps.	Multi-Vit/Min 2 Green Food caps.		Multi-Vit/Min 2 Green Food caps.
Day 10-12		Multi-Vit/Min 2 Green Food caps.	Multi-Vit/Min 2 Green Food caps.	Fatigue Formula	Multi-Vit/Min 2 Green Food caps.
Day 13-15	500 mg tyrosine	Multi-Vit/Min 2 Green Food caps.	Multi-Vit/Min 2 Green Food caps.	Fatigue Formula	Multi-Vit/Min 2 Green Food caps.
Day 16 on	option on day 20, double tyrosine to 1000 mg if not enough energy	Multi-Vit/Min 2 Green Food caps.	Multi-Vit/Min 2 Green Food caps.	Fatigue Formula	Multi-Vit/Min 2 Green Food caps.

Losing It

___ At this stage, it is important to take the properly formulated daily vitamin/mineral supplement to supply your body with abundant nutrients to help restore your adrenal function back to where it used to be.

___ Take the amino acids and herbs that are appropriate for your stage of adrenal burnout.

___ If you are experiencing anxiety, panic attacks, insomnia, and others problems, there are supplements that can help. You may add these supplements to your daily program as needed.

___ Adding power drinks to your daily program is important at this stage.

Losing It	Pre-breakfast	Breakfast	Mid-morning	Lunch	By 3:30 pm	Dinner
Day 1-3		Multi-Vit/Min 2 Green Food caps.				
Day 4-6		Multi-Vit/Min 2 Green Food caps.				Multi-Vit/Min 2 Green Food caps.
Day 7-9		Multi-Vit/Min 2 Green Food caps.		Multi-Vit/Min 2 Green Food caps.		Multi-Vit/Min 2 Green Food caps.
Day 10-12		Multi-Vit/Min 2 Green Food caps.		Multi-Vit/Min 2 Green Food caps.	Fatigue Formula	Multi-Vit/Min 2 Green Food caps.
Day 13-15	500 mg tyrosine	Multi-Vit/Min 2 Green Food caps.	Fatigue Formula	Multi-Vit/Min 2 Green Food caps.	Fatigue Formula	Multi-Vit/Min 2 Green Food caps.
Day 20	option on day 20, double tyrosine to 1000 mg if not enough energy	Multi-Vit/Min 2 Green Food caps.	Fatigue Formula	Multi-Vit/Min 2 Green Food caps.	Fatigue Formula	Multi-Vit/Min 2 Green Food caps.
Day 23	500 to 1000 mg tyrosine	Multi-Vit/Min 2 Green Food caps.	Fatigue Formula	Multi-Vit/Min 2 Green Food caps.	Fatigue Formula	Multi-Vit/Min 2 Green Food caps.
Day 26	500 to 1000 mg tyrosine	Multi-Vit/Min 2 Green Food caps.	Fatigue Formula 500 to 1000 mg tyrosine (optional)	Multi-Vit/Min 2 Green Food caps.	Fatigue Formula	Multi-Vit/Min 2 Green Food caps. 800 mg holy basil

Hitting the Wall

___ Your adrenals are depleted and need nourishment desperately. Take the properly formulated daily vitamin/mineral supplement to supply your body with the nutrients it needs to heal.

____ Power drinks can make a difference in keeping your blood
sugar levels balanced. One a day is a good idea now.

____ Take the amino acids, herbs, and therapeutic nutrients that
are appropriate for your stage of adrenal burnout.

____ You are probably suffering from anxiety, panic attacks, insomnia, and other problems at this stage. There are supplement formulas that can help you and that can be added to
your daily program.

____ It is important to have one to two cups of detox every day.
You can have it anytime you wish.

____ This is a good time to find a health care practitioner who
can evaluate your needs and possibly prescribe natural hydrocortisone.

Hitting the Wall	Pre-breakfast	Breakfast	Mid-morning	Lunch	By 3:30 pm	Dinner	Bedtime or by 10 pm
Day 1-3		Multi-Vit/Min 2 Green Food caps.					100 mg phosphatidylserine
Day 4-6		Multi-Vit/Min 2 Green Food caps.				Multi-Vit/Min 2 Green Food caps.	Increase to 200 mg phosphatidylserine if no improvement in sleep
Day 7-9		Multi-Vit/Min 2 Green Food caps.		Multi-Vit/Min 2 Green Food caps.		Multi-Vit/Min 2 Green Food caps.	100-200 mg phosphatidylserine
Day 10-12		Multi-Vit/Min 2 Green Food caps.		Multi-Vit/Min 2 Green Food caps.	Fatigue Formula	Multi-Vit/Min 2 Green Food caps.	100-200 mg phosphatidylserine
Day 13-15	500 mg tyrosine	Multi-Vit/Min 2 Green Food caps.	Fatigue Formula	Multi-Vit/Min 2 Green Food caps.	Fatigue Formula	Multi-Vit/Min 2 Green Food caps.	100-200 mg phosphatidylserine

Hitting (continued)	Pre-breakfast	Breakfast	Mid-morning	Lunch	By 3:30 pm	Dinner	Bedtime or by 10 pm
Day 20	option on day 20, double tyrosine to 1000 mg if not enough energy	Multi-Vit/Min 2 Green Food caps.	Fatigue Formula	Multi-Vit/Min 2 Green Food caps.	Fatigue Formula	Multi-Vit/Min 2 Green Food caps. 800 mg holy basil	100-200 mg phosphatidyl-serine
Day 23	500 to 1000 mg tyrosine	Multi-Vit/Min 2 Green Food caps.	Fatigue Formula	Multi-Vit/Min 2 Green Food caps. 800 mg holy basil	Fatigue Formula	Multi-Vit/Min 2 Green Food caps. 800 mg holy basil	100-200 mg phosphatidyl-serine
Day 26	500 to 1000 mg tyrosine women: 1-15 mg DHEA men: 1-25 mg DHEA	Multi-Vit/Min 2 Green Food caps.	Fatigue Formula	Multi-Vit/Min 2 Green Food caps. 800 mg holy basil	Fatigue Formula	Multi-Vit/Min 2 Green Food caps. 800 mg holy basil	100-200 mg phosphatidyl-serine
Day 29	500 to 1000 mg tyrosine women: 1-15 mg DHEA men: 1-25 mg DHEA	Multi-Vit/Min 2 Green Food caps.	Fatigue Formula	Multi-Vit/Min 2 Green Food caps. 800 mg holy basil	Fatigue Formula	Multi-Vit/Min 2 Green Food caps. 800 mg holy basil	100-200 mg phosphatidyl-serine
Day 31	500 to 1000 mg Tyrosine women: 1 mg DHEA, increase 1 mg per week, max 15 mg men: 5 mg DHEA increase 1-2 mg per week, max 25 mg	Multi-Vit/Min 2 Green Food caps.	Fatigue Formula 500-1000 mg tyrosine (optional)	Multi-Vit/Min 2 Green Food caps. 800 mg holy basil	Fatigue Formula	Multi-Vit/Min 2 Green Food caps. 800 mg holy basil	100-200 mg phosphatidyl-serine

Burned Out

___ Your body needs all the nourishment you can give it to heal your adrenal glands. Taking the properly formulated daily vitamin/mineral supplement to supply your body with abundant nutrients will be lifesaving at this stage.

___ Sip power drinks made from green food to supply your body with a constant source of nutrients and to keep your blood sugar levels balanced.

___ Take the herbs, therapeutic nutrients, amino acids, and hormones that are appropriate for your stage of adrenal burnout.

___ Add supplement formulas to your daily program to help with your anxiety, panic attacks, and insomnia.

___ It is important to have one to two cups detox tea every day. You can have it anytime you wish.

___ Find a health care practitioner who can evaluate your needs and possibly prescribe natural hydrocortisone.

Burned Out	Pre-breakfast	Breakfast	Mid-morning	Lunch	By 3:30 pm	Dinner	Bedtime or by 10 pm
Day 1-3		Multi-Vit/Min 2 Green Food caps.					100 mg phosphatidylserine
Day 4-6		Multi-Vit/Min 2 Green Food caps.				Multi-Vit/Min 2 Green Food caps.	Increase to 200 mg phosphatidylserine if no improvement in sleep
Day 7-9		Multi-Vit/Min 2 Green Food caps.		Multi-Vit/Min 2 Green Food caps.		Multi-Vit/Min 2 Green Food caps.	100-200 mg phosphatidylserine
Day 10-12		Multi-Vit/Min 2 Green Food caps.		Multi-Vit/Min 2 Green Food caps.	Fatigue Formula	Multi-Vit/Min 2 Green Food caps.	100-200 mg phosphatidylserine

Burned Out (continued)	Pre-breakfast	Breakfast	Mid-morning	Lunch	By 3:30 pm	Dinner	Bedtime or by 10 pm
Day 13-15	500 mg tyrosine	Multi-Vit/Min 2 Green Food caps.	Fatigue Formula	Multi-Vit/Min 2 Green Food caps.	Fatigue Formula	Multi-Vit/Min 2 Green Food caps.	100-200 mg phosphatidyl-serine
Day 20-22	option on day 20, double tyrosine to 1000 mg if not enough energy	Multi-Vit/Min 2 Green Food caps.	Fatigue Formula	Multi-Vit/Min 2 Green Food caps.	Fatigue Formula	Multi-Vit/Min 2 Green Food caps. 800 mg holy basil	100-200 mg phosphatidyl-serine
Day 23-25	500 to 1000 mg tyrosine	Multi-Vit/Min 2 Green Food caps.	Fatigue Formula	Multi-Vit/Min 2 Green Food caps. 500-1000 mg of tyrosine 1/2 hr before lunch	Fatigue Formula	Multi-Vit/Min 2 Green Food caps. 800 mg holy basil	100-200 mg phosphatidyl-serine
Day 26-28	500 to 1000 mg tyrosine	Multi-Vit/Min 2 Green Food caps. 800 mg holy basil	Fatigue Formula	Multi-Vit/Min 2 Green Food caps. 500-1000 mg of tyrosine 1/2 hr before lunch	Fatigue Formula	Multi-Vit/Min 2 Green Food caps. 800 mg holy basil	100-200 mg phosphatidyl-serine
Day 32 on	500 to 1000 mg of tyrosine women: 1 mg DHEA, increase 1 mg per week, max 15 mg men: 5 mg DHEA increase 1-2 mg per week, max 25 mg	Multi-Vit/Min 2 Green Food caps. 800 mg holy basil	Fatigue Formula	Multi-Vit/Min 2 Green Food caps. 500 to 1000 mg of tyrosine 1/2 hr before lunch	Fatigue Formula	Multi-Vit/Min 2 Green Food caps. 800 mg holy basil	100-200 mg phosphatidyl-serine

Simple Solution 7
Oxygenate
Your Body

*Deep breathing improves
your biochemistry and restores
a healthy rhythm to your
nervous system*

Shortcuts to Simple Solution 7

- Defuse your body's fight-or-flight response
by breathing deeply throughout your day—
use cues and reminders to take deep breaths.

- Practice deep breathing exercises when you
can take a break from the action.

---

hances are, as you begin to read this chapter, you
are barely breathing. This may seem like an odd
statement, but it is true that most people do not really *breathe*. Most of
us breathe shallowly, and sometimes we even hold our breath—usually
while gripping the steering wheel of our car.

Breathing is automatic. Deep, healthy breathing, however, is a habit that must be cultivated. Creating a healthy pH in your body helps your autonomic nervous system flow from an uptight sympathetic state into the calming parasympathetic state to aid in digestion, repair, and relaxation. One of the great ways to alkalinize your body is to *breathe deeply*—to literally blow off steam in the form of excess carbon dioxide (CO_2)—an acid that otherwise remains in the body.

Each inhalation brings oxygen into the lungs, while each exhalation expels CO_2. When you draw a breath, oxygen is taken in through your lungs, filtered into your bloodstream, and pumped by your heart into your arteries and then into your capillaries to reach all parts of your body. Cells utilize oxygen in their normal metabolic functioning and create CO_2 as a waste byproduct. The oxygen in your blood is exchanged for CO_2 in your tissues. The blood carrying the CO_2 is then drained back through your veins to your heart and lungs to start the cycle again. With each breath, your red blood cells pick up oxygen and release the CO_2. After being purified of CO_2 and oxygenated, your blood is then pumped back through your heart and into your body.

When you are tense and breathe shallowly or hold your breath, your blood is not being properly purified or oxygenated. CO_2, which is an acidic waste product that is meant to be eliminated, is kept in circulation in your system. This helps create an acid environment in your body. You will find yourself sighing deeply and yawning from lack of oxygen when your body is acidic. This is your body's unconscious wisdom in getting you to blow off the acidic carbon dioxide. Holding your breath, or breathing shallowly is an alarm to your body that you are in danger, signaling your body's sympathetic fight-or-flight response. Practicing deep breathing is a way to help your body move from the uptight sympathetic mode to the calming parasympathetic mode, which contributes to lowering adrenaline and cortisol levels.

The stress hormone adrenaline is secreted from your adrenal glands to protect your body from acute physical and emotional stress. Your adrenals' release of adrenaline is roughly proportional to your brain's perceived intensity of a situation. In other words, the amount and the length of time over which stress hormones are secreted is determined by the degree of danger perceived by your brain. The adrenaline response occurs in the time it takes to snap your fingers.

Imagine that you are relaxing at home after dinner, and it occurs to you that you forgot to take care of an important detail at the office. The telephone rings, and it is your boss asking about the project. In all likelihood, in this fearful or worried situation, you will constrict your breath or breathe shallowly.

You can influence your body's sympathetic adrenaline response in a tense situation like this by taking conscious control and simply breathing deeply and evenly. When you breathe deeply you tell your body: "I am not in danger. I am not fearful." Your brain will send a signal to your adrenals that the time of danger has passed or that the amount of adrenaline secreted is sufficient to deal with the situation. This has two benefits. One, you will then have much more clarity to deal with your situation. Equally important, your adrenals will get a rest from having to churn out adrenaline.

Remember the story of Simon Legree who drove his pickers mercilessly to harvest his orange crop? Throughout the first week the pickers continually harvest and bring Legree many bushels of oranges. The next week Legree is excited by his yield and decides that the pickers should keep on picking all night instead of having dinner and going to bed. So the next week the pickers pick all day and all night without rest or food. That week, they return with a smaller yield. Legree bellows at them that they must continue picking. By the end of the third week, the pickers yield is yet smaller. Legree is panicked now because he needs those oranges, and begins to berate and terrorize the pickers until they finally limp back to work. Exhausted and starving they can only pick a few oranges a day. As the weeks went on, the pickers became so depleted and haggard that they could not even reach up and pick one orange.

This story is a metaphor for what happens to your adrenal glands when your adrenals are constantly called on to work and do not get an opportunity to rest and repair; they will eventually fatigue, affecting all the interconnected systems of the body.

Even if you regularly and intentionally go for the adrenaline rush, by breathing deeply and slowly you can help mediate the amount of adrenaline your adrenals are ordered to secrete. Breathing deeply and slowly will help to spare your adrenals added wear and tear.

Let's say that you are not necessarily going for the adrenaline rush, but you have a job that is chronically stressful. Perhaps you are a newspaper editor who is constantly dealing with deadlines. Maybe you are a teacher, and this year your classroom is filled with unruly kids. When your brain senses greater prolonged stress, cortisol and DHEA are secreted. Again, if your adrenal glands are constantly churning out cortisol and DHEA 24/7 and not given the opportunity to Rest, Repair, or Rejuvenate, their ability to function will diminish. Cortisol production will increase, and DHEA production will decline. You will begin to suffer from insomnia, fatigue, mood swings, low sex drive, weight gain, water retention, and gastrointestinal discomforts, to name a few problems.

By breathing deeply and slowly you can influence your brain so that it will not constantly order your adrenals to secrete the chronic stress hormones cortisol and DHEA.

When you are in an acute or chronically stressful situation, inhale deeply through your nose as if you are actually breathing into your belly. Allow your belly to rise as if it is inflating and feel your chest fill up, your shoulders rise, and your jaw relax. Continue breathing in through your nose and out through your mouth until you feel calm.

Make a mental appointment with yourself. Every time you take a break at work practice a deep breathing exercise for a few minutes or even just a few breaths.

- Sit in a chair, put both feet flat on the floor and get comfortable.

- Close your eyes.

- Rest your hands on your belly, just below your navel.

- Feel the expansion and contraction of your belly as you breathe.

- Take a deep breath as slowly as you can in through your nose, inhaling as fully as possible.

- Fill your lungs all the way up to your shoulders.

- Hold your breath for a second or two, taking one last sniff of air at the top of your lungs.

- Relax your jaw.

- Imagine your tongue is comfortable and limp just lying in the bottom of your mouth.

- Exhale slowly while making the sound of a sigh.

- Repeat this exercise at least five times—or at least once every chance you get.

Another convenient cue is the ringing telephone. Thich Nhat Hanh, one of the world's most beloved Buddhist teachers, suggests that you use the ringing telephone as an opportunity to bring your mind back to the present moment. Set your phone so that it will ring at least four times before your voicemail or answering machine picks up. When you hear your telephone ringing, instead of picking it up immediately, stop for a moment and take a deep, slow breath. Exhale during the silence before the phone rings again. Repeat for a total of three rings before you pick up the phone. Your mind will be focused on what the caller has to say, and your body will be oxygenated from the deep, mindful breathing.

Life is full of stress, and we are not always aware of the tension that creeps into our bodies. I encourage you to place humorous or fun stickers on your wristwatch, or your dashboard or computer or other places you frequently look, to remind yourself to take a couple of deep breaths. Aches and pains can be a reminder to take some deep breaths. If someone in the office bugs you, every time you see that person or hear his or her name, take a huge, deep breath or two. Use whatever cues you can to help you to remember to take relaxing, deep breaths.

I also encourage everyone to take at least five deep, slow breaths before each meal. By exhaling deeply, your body is relieved of some of the acid it has accumulated, therefore calming your nervous system. You nudge your autonomic nervous system back toward balance. When you are in a sympathetic state, peristalsis, the organized, rhythmic muscular contraction of the digestive tract that moves food from the mouth through the digestive system, is slowed down. When you eat while in this state, the food will sit and rot in your digestive tract and is likely to make you sick or constipated or give you diarrhea. Deep breathing allows your body to move to a more parasympathetic state, and your digestive organs can turn on to do their job.

You can live thirty days without food and four days without water, but you can only survive for four minutes without oxygen. Oxygen is truly the source of life—and breathing is within your control.

When a system is out of rhythm, whether it is an assembly line, an engine, or your body, much more energy is expended and much more wear and tear occurs. On the contrary, when a system is in rhythm, it purrs along efficiently. When you breathe short, shallow breaths, you set a staccato rhythm in your body. The goal is to have a peaceful biochemistry that purrs along. When you breathe deeply and slowly you are setting a peaceful rhythm in your body. Breathing

When your body is in sync you will

Feel more pleasure

Find a renewed sense of satisfaction in life

Feel optimistic and positive about life and yourself

Have the energy to enjoy your family again

Remember what made life worth living

Be more likely to accomplish your dreams and goals

Have the energy to enjoy the fruits of your success

Have more self-confidence

Enjoy better relationships

Be able to relax and stop sweating the small stuff

deeply helps you to create order in your chaotic life. In other words, it is one way to take back control of your state of being. Mind and body are not separate. When you slow down the body by breathing deeply, your mind will also begin to slow down. Your thoughts will be crisp and clear, and you are likely to make better decisions, and that will lead to greater success in life.

Simple Solution 7: Oxygenate Your Body
Tailored to your stage of burnout

Driven, Dragging, and Losing It

___ To your brain, your whirlwind life is a constant signal of danger. Holding your breath or breathing shallowly when you are tense sends an alarm to your brain that you are in danger. Instead of allowing your body to shift into a sympathetic adrenaline response in a tense situation, breathe deeply and evenly.

___ It is important for you to do everything you can to prevent the chronic secretion of stress hormones cortisol and DHEA that will wear down your adrenal reserves. Breathing deeply is free. Develop the habit.

___ Make a mental appointment with yourself, or take a break at work to practice a deep breathing exercise for a few minutes or even a few breaths.

___ Use the ringing telephone or other annoying signals as a cue to breathe.

Hitting the Wall and Burned Out

___ Now that you are poised precariously to enter burnout or you have reached burnout, practicing deep breathing can make a big difference in your future health. Your brain has had enough danger signals for ten lifetimes. Begin to influence your body's sympathetic adrenaline response in intense situations by breathing deeply and evenly.

___Your healing prescription includes breathing deeply and slowly throughout the day as well as when you lie down for naps and at bedtime. Breathing deeply and evenly will prevent further damaging secretion of stress hormones cortisol and DHEA.

___Ringing telephones, sitting down to dinner, answering the door, sitting down to read the paper—make mental notes of all the ways you can remember to breathe. Then breathe deeply to heal.

11

Simple Solution 8
Learn About Hidden Toxins

Worse living through chemistry

Shortcuts to Simple Solution 8

- Avoid processed, junk, and fake foods and products that contain chemicals.

- Eat organic foods.

- Avoid water and products containing fluoride.

---

n 1942 Los Alamos, New Mexico, was a top-secret nuclear research site. In 1943, twenty-two-year-old Private Helen Dresher was chosen for her high I.Q. to work with the scientists at the closely guarded military installation there. Helen is a seventy-nine-year-old woman who has a sparkle in her eyes and a tone of command to her voice that belies the years of tragedy and pain she has so gracefully endured. "The military needed people who could help work on calculations that would help develop and produce the atomic bomb," Helen remembered. "The government was testing a variety of radioactive elements at Los Alamos because, at that time, they didn't really know what these elements were good for. They wanted to see if they could serve some purpose in the war. I worked with the scientists in the technical area where there was a machine that was testing what they called the "scatter" (the deflection or disbursement of radioactive particles). They were trying to decide which element they would build the bomb out of. They finally decided on uranium."

During her tenure at the Los Alamos facility, Helen and her colleagues were exposed daily to high levels of radiation. "At that time, scientists did not know the damaging effects of radiation," Helen said. Since so little was known, the military doctors at the facility began to randomly test the personnel. After six months of daily exposure, the doctors began to notice strange and frightening aberrations in Helen's blood cells. She was deployed to a military hospital in another state and was subjected to "every invasive test available at that time."

Helen developed a condition called agranulocytosis (*a gran you low sigh toe sis*), which is the suppression of bone marrow production. Her white blood count was only 1,350—normal is between 5,000 and 10,000. In other words, she had no immune system, which set off a snowball effect of chronic illnesses and conditions. After her discharge from the army the following year, civilian doctors tried innumerable treatments in an attempt to help her, including a protracted course of penicillin. One doctor even removed her spleen, which was thought to be contributing to her low white blood cell count. Removing her spleen did not improve her health, and her illnesses continued. Throughout her life Helen suffered from respiratory infections, allergies, digestive problems, and rheumatoid arthritis. Even more tragic, one of her children was born autistic and legally blind and the second was born legally blind.

Although most of us are not likely to be exposed to as much radiation as Helen was, environmental toxins create a particularly insidious, virulent, and too often invisible form of stress for our bodies. You can be taking one step forward by eating perfectly and exercising and following the Ten Simple Solutions. But if you are ingesting toxins, you are taking many giant steps backward without even knowing it.

Just as Helen was not asked whether or not she would consent to being exposed to radiation, we are part of a universal, involuntary experiment in which we have been and continue to be subjected to hundreds of chemicals, poisons, and toxins already known to be dangerous. These substances are found in everything from baby food to mouthwash. Since toxins are fat soluble, our bodies store toxins from pesticides, chemical food additives, industrial waste, chemicals from cleaning products, air fresheners, and many other sources in our organs and fatty tissues. The human brain, which is 70 percent fat, has become infiltrated with dangerous foreign substances that have never before been included in the chemistry of any living animal. This phenomenon is now being considered as a factor in the development of autism, ADD, ADHD, Parkinson's disease, and Alzheimer's disease.

Environmental poisons damage your liver's ability to detoxify— filter, break down, and eliminate foreign and noxious substances. When your liver is damaged by overexposure to toxins, it can no longer detoxify adequately. Too many toxins then stay in your system and eventually find their way to tissues, cells, and ultimately your genes. Among the damaged cells are those of the immune system. When your immune system is impaired by toxins, your body cannot sufficiently deal with any subsequent toxic exposure, and any subsequent exposure can result in more severe reactions.

Twelve years ago, when Helen was sixty-seven, she had new carpeting installed in her home. "We had to leave the doors and windows closed because it was raining," Helen said. "All of a sudden I could barely walk up to the corner, I was so fatigued. I had inexplicable and very unsettling mood changes, and I felt crazy." Helen was treated at the VA hospital. "They did a sigmoidoscopy [examination of the lower colon] and numerous other invasive tests. I wasn't getting any better and continued feeling disoriented, sick, and tired." As a result of Helen's initial toxic exposure to radiation, her body did not have the reserve to combat this new toxic exposure from the chemicals in her carpeting. Consequently, Helen succumbed to chronic fatigue immune deficiency syndrome, which could not be uncovered by traditional diagnostic procedures.

In a case such as Helen's, the best solution is to immediately eliminate the source of the toxic chemical exposure and then to work on detoxifying the inner system. When Helen came to me she had reached Burned Out and was suffering from chronic fatigue, environmental allergies, atrial fibrillation, severe constipation, and chronic candida. She was determined to feel better. We diligently worked on cleaning up her high-sugar diet. She even gave up her comforting nightly sherry. Through a program that included a rigorous detoxification program, herbs, nutrients, and whole foods, Helen began to recover. At seventy years old, on her own initiative, she began swimming, beginning with barely making it across the pool and eventually swimming thirty laps twice a week. Helen has worked her way back from the Burned Out to the Dragging stage. Just as sixty-year-old Richard Kantor, who began as nearly Burned Out and ended up regaining the musculature of a young man, is my poster boy for recovering from adrenal burnout, Helen is my poster girl. Her tenacity, courage, and determination to recover are inspiring. Having fought humankind's most devastating enemy—radiation—and survived is truly miraculous.

The earth is saturated with poisons, and it is absolutely impossible to avoid exposure. For that reason, it is even more important to build up and support your immune system and make healthy choices when it comes to what you eat and what you allow into your home. When your adrenals are already weak, they cannot appropriately suppress the allergic reactive symptoms caused by toxins (poisons). Often people with toxic damage become increasingly sensitive to the environment in general. Even if your adrenals are healthy, they will eventually be weakened by the long-term exposure to toxins and may even be damaged directly by them, accelerating adrenal burnout.

Most of us harbor sixty to one hundred different toxins in our bodies. These toxins create havoc in numerous debilitating ways. One herbicide could poison cell membranes, a plastic derivative could cause genetic damage, and a pesticide could cause cumulative brain damage like that of Parkinson's disease. Some toxins are known to disable the repair system of our genes and other cellular systems.

Others are known to disarm the immune system. This cumulative damage contributes to the downward spiral of our biochemistry, which ultimately results in such conditions as autoimmune reactions, escalating allergies, chronic fatigue, cancers, Parkinson's disease, and other neurological disorders. In addition to their other dangers, toxic substances are all acid forming and at the very least contribute to an acidic state of sympathetic dominance.

In an interview for this book, David Steinman, a nationally recognized authority on environmental toxins, said: "We know the damaging effects of exposure to pollutants and contaminants in our food, water, air and consumer products. For example, we are chronically exposed to pesticides from home and garden pesticides, food, and water. Even seemingly innocuous products like household cleaners can contain solvents like butyl cellosolve that affect your nervous system. I don't want to make people paranoid—like the legendary ultraenvironmentalist Howard Hughes. On the other hand, it is important to be aware and to be vigilant about the products that we purchase and use."

By avoiding toxins you can

Stop and even reverse accelerated aging

Improve concentration and mental clarity

Have better short-term memory

Have thicker and shinier hair

Have softer and smoother skin with less wrinkles and stronger nails

Lose dark circles under your eyes

To make it easy for you, I offer the following guidelines for avoiding the most common environmental toxins and carcinogens.

Food

Processed, junk, and fake foods contain abundant amounts of sugar and sodium that inhibit satiety and perpetuate cravings. These types of foods also contain toxic chemicals, pesticides, and damaged fats that infuse your body with free radicals. Free radicals damage cells, and damaged cells are more likely to mutate into cancer. Processed, junk, and fake food products *are not real food*—they are dead, devitalized, and deadly. These products lack the building blocks for Repair and Rejuvenation and are acid forming. Eating processed, junk, or fake foods keeps your body in an acidic state of sympathetic dominance. This causes your adrenals to work overtime, which ultimately depletes the adrenal reserve.

The end result of eating these products is fat around your middle, a flabby body, and accelerated aging. Beginning on page 66 are some—but not all—examples of processed, junk, and fake foods to avoid.

Food additives and preservatives have been linked to behavioral disorders, violence, hyperactivity, learning disorders, headaches, irritability, fatigue, ADD, ADHD, and cancer. There are hundreds of food additives and preservatives—aspartame, BHA, BHC, BHT, carrageenan, DHA, lindane, MSG, nitrates, nitrites, potassium bromate, propylene glycol, red dye no. 2, sodium benzoate, sugar, and sulfites are just a few of the common ones. Medical literature is rife with studies that explore, in terrifying detail, the grave dangers of these substances. The safest and healthiest way to approach your diet is, as much as possible, to eliminate additives and preservatives altogether by avoiding processed, fake, and junk foods.

Monosodium glutamate (MSG), a common food additive, is a white crystalline compound used as a flavor enhancer in foods. MSG sensitivity, called the "Chinese restaurant syndrome," can cause skin rash, migraine headaches, severe depression, palpitations, asthma, facial neuralgia, and tight chest—confused with heart pain.

When a product contains 99 percent pure MSG, it is required to be labeled as containing MSG by the FDA. However, smaller amounts of MSG can used without labeling. MSG is in products that list the following ingredients:

Autolyzed yeast
Yeast extract
Hydrolyzed soy protein

Sodium caseinate

Natural flavorings

MSG is found in soups, salad dressings, processed meats, crackers, bread, canned tuna, frozen entrees, ice cream, and frozen yogurt. It is used in low-fat food products to make up for the flavor of the removed fat. To avoid eating MSG it is best not to eat processed, fake, or junk foods.

Nitrates and nitrites are additives that are linked to birth defects and cancer. Because children are smaller, these toxins are even more damaging and dangerous to them.

Rules of thumb to avoid processed, fake, and junk foods

- Eat organic foods whenever possible: meats, dairy, fruits, vegetables, nuts, seeds, and fats.

- When shopping for food, stay on the periphery of your grocery store and avoid the inner aisles where all the fake foods and other toxic chemical products are shelved.

- Shop in stores that specialize in organic, real food.

- Farmer's markets are often a good source of less expensive organic fruits, vegetables, nuts, and eggs.

- Always ask for nitrate-free bacon, hot dogs, and luncheon meats. If you cannot find nitrate-free meats, choose a healthy substitute such as hormone-free turkey breast.

- Before ordering in a restaurant, ask if a dish is prepared with MSG, and if you can have yours made without it. If not, choose another dish.

- To make it simple: do not put anything into your body that is labeled with a long list of chemical gobbledygook.

David Steinman is among the many health authorities who urge people to eat organic foods. "Do eat organic foods as much as possible,"

Steinman said. "If you cannot always buy organic foods, eat healthfully with a good amount of fruits, vegetables, whole grains, legumes and protein sources—especially wild salmon, tuna, and trout which are rich in Omega 3 fatty acids." No matter how hard we try, some processed, junk, and fake food will creep into our diets. Eating high-fiber foods or taking a fiber supplement such as stabilized rice bran will pull some of the toxins out of your body before they are absorbed.

You can find stabilized rice bran at your health food store, or see product recommendations on page 355.

Genetically Manipulated foods

Manufacturers take genetic material (DNA) from one organism or species and put it into another to change the natural characteristics of that organism. For example, scorpion genes have been put into corn to make the plant develop its own insecticide.

We do not yet know the long-term effects that genetic manipulation will have on our health and the health of our environment. Changes in the protein structure of genetically manipulated plants or animals, through the introduction of genetic material, may trigger new allergies and diseases. Many of the genes that are being inserted into food crops have never been part of the human diet. A recent experiment has shown that genetically manipulated foods can, when fed to animals, cause gradual organ and immune system damage.

Perhaps the most ominous example of the genetic manipulation of foods is the soya bean, which is used in over 60 percent of processed foods. Genetic manipulation of the soya bean has been done by the same company that developed Agent Orange during the Vietnam War. The soya bean has been redesigned to be resistant to weedkillers by introducing a sequence of genes that have never been part of the food chain before. It is not known how this new sequence will affect humans.

There is no way tell if a food product contains genetically altered ingredients, since there are no laws that require manufacturers to warn consumers. The best way to avoid these substances is to shop in stores that sell primarily organic foods and to avoid eating processed, junk, and fake foods.

Aspartame and Saccharin

Aspartame has been linked to breast cancer, brain cancer, seizures, neurobehavioral symptoms, headaches, blurred vision, depression, nausea, insomnia, danger to a developing fetus, memory loss, hyperactivity, muscle and joint pain, fatigue, ringing in the ears, diarrhea, and loss of control of limbs.

Saccharin has been studied extensively and linked directly to cancer. The FDA attempted unsuccessfully to ban saccharin ten years ago—and the danger is still there.

Irradiated Food

You read earlier what exposure to radiation did to Helen. Would you eat food grown in Chernobyl? Irradiated food is only one step removed from being exposed to direct radiation. The purpose is to kill pests, eggs, and larvae and to stop ripening and sprouting to lengthen the shelf life of foods. Irradiation exposes foods to a high level of gamma radiation. *The source of this radiation is nuclear waste.*

Irradiation has been linked to a dramatic increase in free radicals in the body, cataracts, reduced fertility, testicular tumors, kidney damage, premature aging, and death.

Irradiated foods are required by the FDA to be labeled with an internationally recognized symbol known as the "radura"—that looks like a flower logo—as well as the statement: "Treated with ionizing radiation."

Many spices are irradiated. Nonirradiated lines of spices are produced by Spice Hunter, McFadden Farm, and Spice Garden. You will probably find more brands at your health food store.

Peanuts

If you love peanut butter, be aware that peanuts grow a carcinogenic mold called aflatoxin. Look for products that are certified "aflatoxin free." Wild Oats makes an aflatoxin-free organic peanut butter.

Household Products

We all would like to feel that we can use laundry detergent, hairspray, and all the other products we are accustomed to using and have the outcome be as sunny as a television commercial. The truth is that most toxic household products contain harmful, even carcinogenic toxins. Long-term exposure to household products can result in lung cancer and/or damage to the liver, kidneys, and central nervous system.

Petrochemicals are made from gasoline byproducts that are harmful to health. Avoiding petrochemicals, such as mineral oil and Vaseline, diminishes your exposure to gasoline byproducts, which are known carcinogens.

Many people have not investigated using natural, biodegradable, chemical-free, environmentally safe products because they assume that they are too expensive. It is true that when these products first came onto the market they were much higher priced then the standard fare. As more people are using these products, however, the prices have dropped. I encourage you to support these safe and healthy industries by using these products.

If you are buying the following products from a large chain grocery or drug store, they are likely too toxic for you to be using at any of the five stages of adrenal burnout:

> Antiperspirants containing aluminum
> Cosmetics
> Laundry detergent, household, and garden supplies
> Moisturizing products containing petrochemicals
> Pet products
> Self-care products
> Toothpaste with fluoride

This information is not meant to make you worry or stress out. You can make significant changes by taking small steps, such as switching to an aluminum-free deodorant and using a toothpaste that does not contain fluoride. If your local stores do not stock environmentally safe products, they can be purchased through mail-order catalogs. Some are listed on page 356.

Electropollution resulting from electromotive forces (EMFs), for example extremely low-frequency fields (ELFs), is a problem that has grown exponentially over the past one hundred years.

Electricity is the phenomenon arising from the existence of charge. Most elementary particles of matter possess charge, either positive or negative. Two particles of like charge, both positive or both negative, repel each other; two particles of unlike charge are attracted. Alternating current (AC) is a flow that repeats in a cycle. The number of repetitions of the cycle occurring each second is defined as the frequency, which is expressed in Hertz (Hz). The frequency of ordinary household current in the United States is sixty cycles per second (60 Hz). The frequency of the human brain runs one to two cycles of AC per second while sleeping or resting and eighteen to twenty-two cycles per second when using intense mental concentration. The electromagnetic frequencies of televisions, microwaves, electric blankets, hair dryers, computers, cell telephones, radios, and all of the appliances and electrical devices in our environment are not compatible with human cellular function. The current from these appliances disrupts a healthy human electrical current and can actually cause cellular mutation.

Extremely low-frequency fields are one of the contributing factors to electropollution. ELFs affect people in their own households, where ELF wave–emitting devices, for example, televisions, fluorescent lights, electric blankets, microwave ovens, are present. A two-year Environmental Protection Agency (EPA) study recommended that ELF fields be classified as "probable human carcinogens" alongside chemical toxins such as PCBs, formaldehyde, and dioxin.

To avoid some electromagnetic pollution

- Use a headset or an earpiece with your cell phone.

- Do not use electric blankets or heating pads.

- Stay as far as possible from outside electrical poles and transformers.

- Stay at least three feet away from electrical devices such as TV, radio, video, bedside clocks, and microwaves.

- Stay three feet away from electric wall plugs when sleeping, as they emanate an electric field if something is plugged in.

- Unplug waterbeds when you go to sleep.

- Use negative magnetic field therapy, described on page 140.

Silver fillings

For one hundred and fifty years silver fillings have been used by dentists: a silver amalgam that contains fifty percent mercury. It is well documented that mercury poisoning can cause myriad illnesses. A review of studies on mercury toxicity concluded that mercury dental fillings are the major contributing source of the presence of mercury in humans. Researchers have been seriously looking at the role mercury dental fillings play in the development of Alzheimer's disease, multiple sclerosis, Parkinson's disease, and other progressive degenerative diseases. Scientists are also looking at the link between chronic and/or unexplained illnesses and the presence of mercury in the body. The presence of mercury in your body can damage your brain, heart, lungs, liver, kidney, blood cells, and hormones and cause hair loss, fatigue, and enzyme abnormalities as well as suppress your body's immune system.

Silver fillings are being banned around the world. Dentists are required by law to dispose of the silver fillings they remove as hazardous material. If you are suffering from an untreatable illness, it is in your best interest to have your hair tested or your urine tested to find out the level of toxic metals, including mercury, in your system. If your levels are high, you may find relief from many of your symptoms by having your silver fillings removed. There are dentists who are trained and experienced in removing silver fillings so that your body is not further contaminated by the heavy metal. Once your fillings are removed, chelation can rid your body of the rest of the heavy metals.

Mercury is not the only heavy metal that can accumulate in your system. Lead, aluminum, and cadmium are three other common toxins. These heavy metals exist in the food chain, water, air, and self-care and household products as well as coming from industrial sources. The presence of heavy metal in your system can cause symptoms that cannot be ascribed to a particular condition or disease.

Symptoms of heavy metal toxicity

Burning sensation on tongue
Cold hands and feet, even in
    moderate or warm weather
Constipation
Diarrhea
Difficulty making simple
    decisions
Facial twitching or twitching
    of other muscles
Faulty memory
Feeling bloated
Feeling itchy
Feeling out of breath
Fluid retention
Frequent urination at night
Hair loss
Headaches after eating
Heartburn

Insomnia
Irritability
Joint pain
Jumpiness/nervousness
Leg cramps
Metallic taste in mouth
Numbness and tingling in
    extremities
Ongoing depression
Ringing in ears
Sudden, unexplained, or un-
    solicited anger/rage
Tachycardia
Tremors or shakiness
Unexplained chest pain
Unexplained chronic fatigue
Unexplained rashes and/or
    skin irritation

Hair analysis is a noninvasive, inexpensive screening test that can be done without a doctor's order. Hair analysis will tell you if you have high levels of heavy metals such as lead, aluminum, cadmium, and mercury. There are numerous papers on the accuracy and efficacy of hair testing, particularly for toxic metals such as mercury. The EPA published an authoritative study in 1979 in which more than four hundred reports on hair testing were reviewed. The authors concluded that hair is a "meaningful and representative tissue for biological monitoring of most of the toxic metals."

The lab I recommend for hair analysis is:

Great Smokies Diagnostic Laboratory
63 Zillicoa St.
Asheville, NC 28801
800 522-4762
http://www.gsdl.com

Once you know if you have high levels of heavy metals in your system, you can rid your body of them through chelation. A chelating agent is a compound that binds with heavy metals, pulls them from your tissue, and carries them from your body via your urine and stool. Ethylenediaminetetraacetic acid (*eth el een die amean tetra a see dik*) (EDTA) is the most traditional and well-documented method of chelation. EDTA was first used during World War II in an attempt to purge soldiers of the nerve gases they were exposed to on the battlefield. In addition to leaching toxic heavy metals from your body, EDTA has many other benefits, including the ability to open up blood vessels in people at risk for heart disease by pulling calcium deposits (plaque) out of arteries.

Intravenous chelation therapy is done in a doctor's office and takes several hours. Chelation can pull out the good with the bad, so extra mineral replacements are required the day of treatment and the day after.

I am excited that we can use something orally now for chelation. Another chelating agent, meso 2, 3-dimercaptosuccinic acid (*die mer kap toe suck sin ik*) (DMSA), under the brand name Chemet, can be taken in pill form. The typical protocol I use for an adult is a maximum of 300 milligrams a day for five days, then taking three weeks off, and repeating this process until the person's test is clear of heavy metals. I will have the same test repeated after six months because heavy metals can emerge over time from deep stores within the body. DMSA crosses the blood-brain barrier better than intravenous EDTA, so it very effectively reduces lead and mercury found in the brain.

Chemet and EDTA are both prescription drugs that can only be obtained through a doctor. Since all doctors are not versed in chelation therapy, I recommend you find a doctor who is trained in this area.

If you have symptoms of heavy metal exposure, or if you live in an old building with old pipes, paint, and/or asbestos, or if you live or work near an industrial plant, you may have been exposed to heavy metals or concentrated toxins. If you suspect heavy metal poisoning, seek the treatment of a physician who is trained and knowledgeable about toxins and chelation therapy. For more information on chelation therapy and physician referrals contact this agency:

American College for Advancement in Medicine
P.O. Box 3427
Laguna Hills, CA 92654
(800) 532-3688 or (964) 583-7666
www.acam.org

The herb cilantro is a natural mercury chelator. Cilantro can reach the deep mercury stores, including those in your brain, and leach it from your system. I encourage all of my patients who have silver fillings and any signs of mercury toxicity to eat one tablespoon of chopped cilantro every day.

Enteric-coated enzymes are a milder form of chelation that are taken orally. They are released not in the stomach, but in the small intestine, where they are absorbed into the bloodstream. When these enzymes are taken between meals, they break down abnormal connective tissue, which improves the circulation to cells and cellular function, which in turn gives the body better access to all the nutrients coming in. Sea algae in green food are natural heavy metal chelators.

A Simple Detox Day

A detox day is one way for you to pay valuable attention to yourself. By detoxifying, after very little effort you can see some immediate results in the way you look and feel. Many people end up losing significant amounts of weight during a detox without even trying. You can indulge yourself in detox as often as you want.

- Eat only organic foods—especially on detox days.

- Take 25 to 500 milligrams of niacin, which helps to release toxins. If you experience a hot flush from the niacin, this is normal and not dangerous.

- To enhance detoxification, engage in some form of aerobic exercise for twenty to thirty minutes to increase your heart rate to a moderate working level. Exercise at your level of fitness. If you are not used to vigorous exercise, walk at a fast pace.

- Sit in a sauna, set at approximately 140 degrees, for up to thirty minutes—some people will only tolerate the heat for five minutes. Even low-heat saunas can help to detoxify the body of a lifetime of pollutants and contaminants.

- Drink eight to twelve glasses of water or detox tea throughout your detox day.

- Drink a super green food power drink the morning of your detox. Green foods are detoxing and chelating—they actually pull out heavy metals from your system. Recipes can be found on pages 334–339.

Detox

Supplement Formula to Take on Detox Day

Many chemical substances are referred to as xenohormones (*zeeno hormones*)—molecules that exert hormonal influences in your body. Most xenohormones act like estrogen, which is a growth factor. The estrogen-like effects of xenohormones are thought to be a major contributing factor to the alarming rise in cancers. In addition, hormones are your body's communication system. An overabundance of any hormone upsets the balance and results in illness and disease. I recommend a detox formula designed to selectively protect the organs, such as the prostate, breast, and uterus, that are most vulnerable to stress, toxins, and the damaging effects of xenohormones. You can take this formula in addition to your everyday supplement formula.

> 200 milligrams green tea leaf extract
> 500 milligrams D-limonene oil
> 2.5 milligrams lycopene
> 50 milligrams turmeric rhizome extract
> and an Ayurvedic blend of herbs including hellebore root, spreading hog weed, andrographis aerial parts, chicory seed, ginger rhizome, amala fruit, Indian gall fruit, long pepper fruit, embelia fruit, phyllanthus, trailing eclipta leaf and root, and arjuna myrobalan bark.

Take this list to your health food store and match it as closely as possible. Product recommendations are listed on page 355.

Constipation

In nature all animals have a bowel movement after they eat. In my opinion moving your bowels once a day is the bare minimum. During detox it is more critical that your bowels move every day to flush out the toxins you are trying to eliminate. If you are constipated, the toxins will sit in your intestines, and some will be reabsorbed. At the same time, you do not want to induce diarrhea. The food and nutrients you eat must remain in your intestinal tract long enough to be properly absorbed. When you flush food out too fast, you become nutrient deficient.

Irritating laxatives such as cascara sagrada, which is a primary ingredient in many laxative formulas, can have long-term damaging effects on your colon. Instead, increase fiber in your diet by eating fruit, vegetables, nuts, rice bran, and whole grains—the fiber attracts the toxins and pulls them out of your body before they can be reabsorbed or recycled. Or take the following constipation formula.

Formula to Relieve Constipation

Take at bedtime. Begin with 200 milligrams magnesium oxide or magnesium citrate—you may increase the dosage in 200 milligram increments until your bowels move regularly. The dose for magnesium is very individual, so begin low and increase the dosage as needed. Reduce the dosage if you experience loose bowels. Unlike irritating laxatives, magnesium does not create laxative dependency. You may find magnesium citrate at your health food store.

Take one eight-ounce glass of detox tea or water.

You can find detox teas in any health food store. Look for teas that contain a combination of dandelion, burdock, alfalfa, red clover, slippery elm, goldenseal, and silymarin (milk thistle).

Water, which is the principal constituent of all body fluids, is essential for detoxification. During detox, drink a lot of clean water or good, naturally caffeine-free herb tea. Four to eight glasses a day are essential for good health.

This is a lot of information to absorb. Again, my intention is not to make you worry or stress out. Begin with small changes. Do only what you feel comfortable doing. The goal is to incorporate the Ten Simple Solutions one small step at a time so that each step is a source of good health, not more stress.

Simple Solution 8: Learn About Hidden Toxins
Tailored to your stage of burnout

Driven, Dragging, and Losing It

___ To protect your immune system, begin to make healthy choices when it comes to what you eat and what you allow into your home.

___ Avoid processed, junk, and fake foods—anything that has a label with a long list of chemical gobbledygook.

___ Eat organic foods whenever possible.

___ Avoid household and self-care products that contain harmful chemicals.

___ Use safe and healthy products from your health food store or catalogs.

___ Avoid products and water containing fluoride.

___ Do what you can to stay away from electropollution.

___ Consider having your silver fillings removed by a dentist experienced in this procedure.

___ If you have symptoms of heavy metal toxicity, have your hair analyzed, and if you have high levels of heavy metals in your system, see a doctor trained in chelation. References are on page 260.

___ Practice regular detoxification.

If you are in the Driven, Dragging, and Losing It stages and want to be really safe, follow the guideline for Burned Out.

Hitting the Wall and Burned Out

___ At these stages chemical exposure could mean the difference between life and early death. To restore adrenal function and to rebuild your immune system, it is crucial to make healthy choices when it comes to what you eat and what you allow into your home.

___ Giving up processed, junk, and fake foods—anything that has a label with a long list of chemical gobbledygook—could mean the difference in your recovery.

___ Organic foods are more expensive, but they are not nearly as dear as your life. Organic foods will heal you and protect you from further toxic exposure.

___ Clean out your cupboards and get rid of all the household cleaning products, air fresheners, poisons, and garden supplies that contain harmful chemicals. There are plenty of safe and affordable products on the market today.

___ Purge your bathroom closets and drawers of unhealthy self-care products. Health food stores and catalogs carry nurturing alternatives.

___ Drink bottled water to avoid chemicals and fluoride. Toss the fluoride toothpaste and use a natural alternative.

___ Do what you can to stay away from electropollution.

___ When you feel strong enough, consider having your silver fillings removed by a dentist experienced in this procedure.

___ If you have symptoms of heavy metal toxicity, have your hair analyzed and if you have high levels of heavy metals in your system, rid your body of heavy metals through chelation. See page 260 for doctors trained in chelation.

___ Practicing regular detoxification will help you heal faster now.

Simple Solution 9
Have Fun
Every Day

Are you having fun yet?

Shortcuts to Simple Solution 9

- Take steps to make your life more enjoyable.

- Get off the treadmill and be more spontaneous.

- Associate with positive people.

The busy schedule is a perfect setup for creating unhealthy neurotransmitters. Since our neurotransmitters determine our future well-being, one way to insure an ongoing healthy supply is to have some fun every day. I understand that life is stressful and busy no matter how your schedule shakes out—and that it might not be that easy to find the time for fun every day. That is why I encourage you to have a new attitude toward having fun. Imagine fun more as a state of mind than a time-consuming activity. Sure, activities such as downhill skiing, knitting, playing cards, horseback riding, dancing, bowling, even watching the Super Bowl on TV are great examples of fun. But they are only one category of fun. When I say "Have fun," I am not necessarily talking about dropping everything and going to the movies. I am also *not* talking about experiences like binge drinking or partying or obsessive exercise that wreak havoc on your adrenals and your life. Fun activities improve your life at no cost to your health. I am talking about having experiences, however fleeting, that take you out of the trials and tribulations of daily life, that absorb you so that your mind is cleared of concerns and your body and mind are united and uplifted—even momentarily.

Even short periods of fun during our day will leave us more relaxed and hopeful, with sharper senses; more open to ideas and more creative; more generous to ourselves and to others; and more spontaneous. The high that we get from having fun can renew our flagging spirits and recharge us in ways that manmade drugs cannot. Philosophers, politicians, and comedians have long recognized that anything that gets us to smile and laugh acts as a balm to recharge our efforts and bring us closer to one another.

Through research efforts in the field of psychoneuroimmunology (PNI), we now have solid evidence that humor and laughter can change our biochemistry. Laughter and having fun create healthy neurotransmitters, which in turn produce and perpetuate feelings of happiness and joy. Increasingly, studies are demonstrating that laughter and humor boost immunity, diminish pain, and help people deal with the stress of life. Dr. Aristo Wojdani, director of the Immunosciences Laboratory in Los Angeles, commented: "Positive and negative experiences affect your immune system. Stressful, sad and scary experiences have been shown to suppress immune function for twenty-hours after the experience. On the other hand, fun, enjoyable experiences boost the immune system's function for three days after the fun experience." This means that just a few fun experiences a week can give you a consistently stronger immune system and improve your health.

To recover from adrenal burnout and to begin rebuilding adrenal reserve, you need to find ways to either avoid or cope with situations that keep you in a sympathetic-dominant state. Having fun, laughing, and getting pleasure from your tasks, family, and friends helps free your body from the grasp of sympathetic dominance.

Behaviors that lead to sympathetic dominance

Skipping meals/dieting

Eating processed, junk, or fake foods

Not exercising or exercising too much

Avoiding or neglecting relaxation and other ways to calm your central nervous system

Blowing past your own fatigue to finish the day's work

Not getting enough sleep

Using sugar, caffeine, nicotine, drugs, or herbal stimulants to function at a higher rate when you are already tired

Breathing shallowly when tense, instead of breathing deeply

Exposing yourself to toxins through the environment, household products, and food

Worrying

Mentally replaying stressful inner dialogues

Neglecting fun and relaxing activities that allow you to clear your mind

Putting yourself last

Ideally, you want to reduce prolonged exposure to situations where you experience great physical and emotional demands—uncertainty, threat, fear, panic, worrying dependence, defensiveness—or experiences that keep you in a heightened sense of readiness. Of course, given the jobs and living situations we have chosen, it is not always possible to remove ourselves from these stressors. Sometimes we have to develop ways of deflecting these harmful influences, including developing a strong sense of humor to cope with them.

Unpressured, relaxed, and humorous moments signal your body that the time of danger is over and allow your parasympathetic state to emerge. It has been shown that those pesky stress hormones that keep you in a sympathetic-dominant state can be lowered by having a few good laughs. In other words, having fun can nudge your autonomic nervous system to flow from the sympathetic to the parasympathetic state, create healthy neurotransmitters, boost serotonin levels, and foster a well-tuned, rhythmic biochemistry. When you do not make time for fun, when you take yourself and your life too seriously and do not stop to enjoy experiences, you create unhealthy neurotransmitters that contribute to panic biochemistry.

Panic biochemistry occurs when we repeat or are caught in behaviors that keep us in a state of sympathetic dominance. The state of sympathetic dominance uses up your calming neurotransmitters that keep you on an even keel. As these neurotransmitters are depleted, you can become agitated and more easily pushed over the edge. Every little thing becomes a big deal. Taking time to have fun in your life creates healthy, calming neurotransmitters that will help you buffer the effects of toxins, lower the stress on your adrenals, and reduce the damage to your metabolism and nervous system caused by overproduction of the stress hormones cortisol and adrenaline.

Strategies for Having Fun

Many approaches and activities can lead you to the state of mind called fun. I encourage you to start with the one strategy of those discussed here that seems the easiest and most natural for you. If I could write a prescription for you it would read: "Have fun two to seven days per week."

Having fun is different for everyone. What one person thinks is fun, another might think is drudgery. Whatever you do for stress release and fun needs to be something that makes you feel good. I asked a few people to place activities they consider fun after the descriptions of the fun strategies. Seeing what other people find fun may help you recognize the fun you already have in your life.

Take Fun Breaks

You can take fun breaks during the day, even if it is five minutes to talk to someone on the phone with whom you share private jokes.

You can both schedule breaks and be open to spontaneous breaks. Go to lunch with a friend, read the comics, listen to your favorite drive-time radio program, spend fifteen minutes in your garden or with your cat or dog. Taking a fun break helps elevate your serotonin so that you do not have to reach for a candy bar at 3 P.M. Especially when you are having a craving, try thinking of something fun and stress-releasing that you can do for five or ten minutes. Here are a few real-life examples from men and women:

- Listening to National Public Radio and reading the newspaper.

- I love my work, so most of my day is fun.

- Playing video games.

- My husband and I go out dancing. We do our own dance, which is a mixture of swing and lambada—that is the most fun thing in the world.

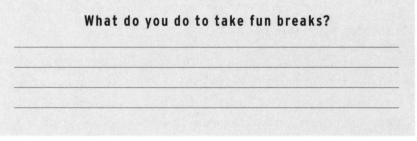

What do you do to take fun breaks?

Stop and Smell the Roses

When you stop and smell the roses, you recognize the fun moments that are already in your life. We all have the tendency to rush, so even our enjoyable moments become a blur. This is never more evident than when trying to enjoy your own wedding. I do not know one woman who remembers any of the details of her wedding ceremony or reception. Thanks to cameras and video equipment, we can enjoy the party in retrospect. My favorite technique to help you here is to establish a daily ritual to mention your fun or meaningful daily moments to a friend, your spouse or partner, in your journal, or in your prayers.

Having fun means finding enjoyment and pleasure in the life you are already leading. Ask yourself, does it have to be so stressful? Perhaps you are making your life more complicated than it needs to be. When you recognize and acknowledge the fun you already have in your life, you will feel less stressed. Here are a few real-life examples from men and women:

- I pray at least once a day to thank God for what I have in my life and to ask for guidance.

- I rearrange furniture and come up with new decorating ideas. When I get connected to my home, it allows me to stop, to connect with my life, and to appreciate my life and blessings.

- I don't have a gardener—it's all me. So getting my hands in the dirt makes me appreciate my beautiful garden.

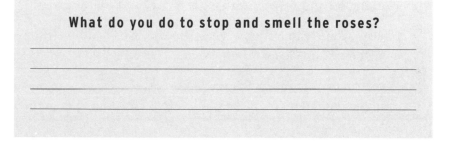

What do you do to stop and smell the roses?

Schedule Activities That Relax and Uplift You

Most Driven people's lives are dictated by their calendars. They first create the commitments that structure their lives, and then they work like crazy to meet their obligations. All of us can make time for one or a few activities a week that we know will bring us some enjoyment and will be good for our adrenal health. Some of us are able to set aside a day a week for golf. Most of us have to settle for fewer and shorter activities. Since your health and happiness are priorities to you, schedule in at least one activity a week and then follow through on it. I have found that having a couple of partners who enjoy the same activity can help Driven people live up to their obligation to have fun.

The idea here is to schedule activities for the pure sake of having fun, not to further your career or to make you or your family more popular. Your fun activities are supposed to make you *feel* better. Whatever activities you choose—going to the movies, playing tennis, baking cookies with your kids—do them because they make you feel better, not just because they make you look better, satisfy other people's wants or needs, or promote your career. In other words, if you would get more satisfaction on a Saturday morning by staying home and washing your car than going off to play golf with someone from work, then washing your car is the healthy and wise choice. But please do not wash your car just because you want your neighbors to admire it. This time is for *you*. Here are a few real-life examples from men and women:

- Working on my property with my chainsaw and splitting logs.

- I make a date with a friend to shop—especially at sales—then I come home and clean out my closet.

- I live on a mountaintop. For the last twenty-six years I have had a standing date to meet my neighbor every morning and go on a hike.

What activities do you schedule that relax and uplift you?

_____

_____

_____

_____

Make Your Life More Spontaneous

We all get set in routines and trudge along the conveyor belt of our days. The most stress-releasing and fun moments in life often spring from spontaneity. It is difficult to build spontaneity into a highly structured life. Most of us look forward to retirement so that we can free ourselves from major obligations and live our lives more moment to moment, doing what we want. I encourage you not to wait until retirement to allow your life to be more spontaneous. Finding a few minutes here or there for fun is one way to break the drudgery and be spontaneous. Here are a few real-life examples from men and women:

- I work at home. Once in a while my dogs will get fed up with my work and will talk me into going to the beach, so I drop everything and take them.

- I take a spontaneous day off work, go out to lunch, and have a glass of wine.

- My husband and I regularly take trips. We don't take tours or schedule any agendas. We meet strangers and sit and talk for hours to find out about them.

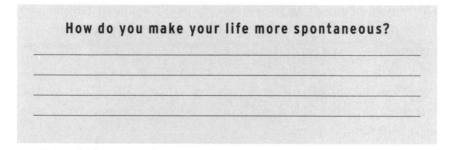

How do you make your life more spontaneous?

Treating Yourself as an Honored Guest

Remember how Mom always took the burned piece of toast? Martyrs have a special place in history but generally do not make for very happy, fun people. Treat yourself like an honored guest on a regular basis. Day spas are opening up all over the country. Take a day off and get pampered. Buy yourself something that you have always wanted. Be as nice to yourself as you would be to other people. Here are a few real-life examples from men and women:

- I ask someone to help me out when I need it instead of trying to be the hero.

- I have a facial, manicure, pedicure, or massage or all four.

- I treat myself to a new outfit. I think I deserve to have something nice once in awhile.

How do you treat yourself as an honored guest?

_____

_____

_____

_____

Associate with Positive People

We have all heard about people in dire circumstances—people who are undergoing chemotherapy, for example, who inspire others with their positive, even joyful attitudes. Then there are those who really have nothing to complain about but who manage to bring you down with their moaning the moment they enter the room. Moaners typically want others to absorb their negativity and to commiserate with their complaints about life.

Unfortunately, some people have moaners in their family whom they cannot completely avoid. In that case, the best approach is to try to set a positive example and not to get sucked in by the complaining.

Do what you can to work around and socialize with positive, fun-loving, appreciative people. The aim is not only to hear affirming messages more of the time but also to be appreciated when you are positive. Positive companions can do a lot to counteract the stresses of life. Here are a few real-life examples from men and women:

- I call my two partners who live in other cities who buoy me up.

- I review my day with my wife, who gives me encouragement.

- I play with my dogs—they are the most positive people I know.

- I avoid negative people. My rule is that I will listen to any amount of complaining as long as someone is doing something about the problem. The moment it becomes a tape that is played just so the person can hear themselves talk, I avoid that person.

- I had plenty of years when my first marriage was positive. When I split up with my ex-husband, it had become like the dark night of the soul. So it was time to leave that. Now my life is more positive, and my relationship with my husband is the most positive influence in my life.

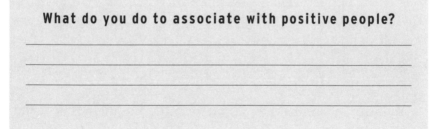

What do you do to associate with positive people?

Be Positive

When you associate with positive people and have a purpose in your life, you are likely to be more positive yourself. Despite life's roadblocks, keep your sights focused on reachable goals. Give yourself credit when you achieve a goal, no matter how small it seems. Regrets and fretting over mistakes and failures only waste your precious resources. Now is a good time to acknowledge your mistakes. Then you can move forward in your life. You can influence your biochemistry with thoughts and actions that create healthy neurotransmitters. Your mental and adrenal health depend on your ability to keep your head up and keep smiling. If you recognize your own negativity, perhaps looking at your psychogene can help you understand where this negativity comes from and this time, as an adult, choose new beliefs that serve you better.

What is your psychogene equation?

_____→ led to

What is your psychogene—your beliefs and fears?

_____→ led to

What emotion can you identify with your psychogene?

_____→ led to

What behaviors have you developed in an attempt to appease that emotion?

_____

What emotional or physical symptoms have you developed as a result?

You may believe that life has no meaning and there is no hope. This type of psychogene will tarnish all areas of your life. Beliefs are a choice, and you can make new choices that will support and carry you in your future. Practice is the best way you can make changes from negative to affirmative thinking. Make a commitment to yourself to write down negative thought and beliefs that flit through your mind. Next to each negative thought, write a positive counterthought. When negative thoughts arise, remember your list, and counter with a positive thought. In time, you will naturally make healthy neurotransmitters that will change you from a negative to a positive person. Make photocopies of this page or write in a journal.

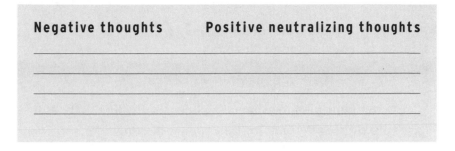

Negative thoughts   **Positive neutralizing thoughts**

Here are a few real-life examples from men and women on how to stay positive:

- I remind myself fairly often that most people are trying to be responsible.

- To avoid negativity I remember clearly how difficult my life was when I was younger, and I appreciate daily all that I have and all that I have accomplished.

- When I get into situations when my emotions start to swing inappropriately, I am learning to stop reacting from old tendencies. I'm working on learning how to stop little emotional disasters from happening. My challenge is to stay positive by not getting beaten down by little things.

What do you do to be positive?

Simple Solution 9: Have Fun Every Day
Tailored to your stage of burnout

Driven, Dragging, and Losing It

___ If you want to enjoy your life when you finally fulfill all of your dreams, develop the habit of having fun.

___ If you develop the habit of stopping to smell the roses today, years from now you will not look back and wonder where your life went.

___ Even though your ambition rules you, take the time to schedule activities that relax and uplift you. Your productive years will last longer.

___ Avoid falling into the treadmill trap by making your life more spontaneous.

___ Even though your life is scheduled to the hilt, treat yourself as an honored guest from time to time.

___ Developing the habit of associating with positive people will further your dreams.

___ It is hard to be driven and be negative at the same time. Make a pact with yourself to stay positive.

Hitting the Wall and Burned Out

___ Maybe you no longer believe that life is a bowl of cherries. Why slip any deeper toward ill health and negativity when some very simple solutions like having fun every day can help you recover?

___ You have come this far without stopping. You have probably accomplished some of your goals. Stop and smell the roses now. There is nothing like basking in your own glory and rewards. You deserve it.

___ There is nothing stopping you from babying yourself. Schedule activities that relax and uplift you now.

___ Allow yourself to be a little more spontaneous. No one is going to think you are slacking.

___ A massage can work wonders. Give yourself a fresh perspective every once in a while by treating yourself as an honored guest.

___ Now that you are so close to burnout or you are burned out, do you really want to associate with negative people? No one is keeping you in those relationships but yourself. Make more time to be with those who uplift you.

___ Remember when you were positive about yourself and about life? You can recultivate that spirit now. Staying positive is a powerful force. When you feel negativity creeping in, let it go and replace it with a positive thought.

Simple Solution 10
Cultivate
SELF-fulfillment

*You really do have a choice in
how your life is going to be lived*

Shortcuts to Simple Solution 10

• Do unto yourSELF as you would do unto others.

• Learn to say no.

• Delete your SHOULDS and face off
with your beast of never enough.

On November 3, 1993, black mushrooms of smoke, like detonated bombs, loomed incongruously over the tranquil blue water of the Pacific Ocean off the coast of Malibu, California. The sky snowed ash as a 2,000-degree firestorm, fueled by seventy-mile-an-hour Santa Ana winds, blew furiously over the foothills toward the sea. In the next thirty-six hours, one hundred homes were incinerated. Fifty-one-year-old Whitney Bonnard and her husband were among the thousands of residents ordered to evacuate the area by sheriffs' helicopters. The Bonnards were renting and had decided it was not necessary to carry fire insurance. The fire consumed everything they owned.

The coals were still smoldering when Whitney went full tilt into trying to put her life back together. "Whatever I do, I'm always very involved—whether it's my family or my church or my interior design business. But after the fire, everything just sped up." Her commitments tripled as she attempted to pull her weight, first by replacing the bare essentials of their home and then trying to earn and save enough money to recreate their former life.

In addition to taking every design job that came along, Whitney continued to be devoted to her husband, children, and grandchildren, as well as teaching design and Bible study. Four years after the fire, Whitney was still going strong. "I didn't think I had a choice about how hard I had to work to regroup after the fire. I was still acting like I was twenty-five instead of fifty-five. One night I was sick with the flu, but I was working on putting together a baby shower for a dear friend, so I didn't slow down. I was dehydrated and hadn't eaten all day. I passed out and ended up in the hospital."

The Yes Person

With strawberry-blonde curls and a perpetual smile, Whitney is an outwardly and inwardly beautiful soul. Whitney is the person that you want on your team—the person who will spend every ounce of who she is making sure everything gets done. As is the case for many people who put themselves last, her drive and constant inner conflict had led to hypertension.

When Whitney came to see me, I took one look at her and said, "If you keep going like this you will end up in the hospital with much more serious problems. You need to stop, look around, and reorder your priorities. Do nothing for thirty days. Tell everyone 'no,' and if they give you any problems tell them to call your doctor." Before she left my office, we practiced saying no together and had a good laugh over it.

It slowly began to dawn on Whitney that the fire had uncovered a number of issues that she had never been aware of before. "I come from a very controlling family. My attitude had always been, I'll do it. I can control it. I can make it happen faster or better if I do it myself. I just never realized how controlling I was. I made up my mind then and there that I didn't want to be that person."

Learning to Say No

Whitney's psychogene was that she had to take care of everyone else's needs to be valued, and her fear of not doing enough → led to denial about her own needs and vulnerabilities → led to trying to please everyone at the expense of her health → led to hypertension and exhaustion.

For Whitney, wanting to change was a start. At first it was "very uncomfortable" to do nothing. "Friends would want to get together for lunch and I would say, 'You know, I really can't do that, but if you would like to come and sit with me or walk with me on the beach that would be lovely.' After I did my thirty days, I really liked it. I saw the benefits, so now I try to take a couple a days out of the week where I really have nothing scheduled and go with whatever is going to happen in that day."

It is interesting to note that Whitney's choice of words, "I did my thirty days," sounds more like a description of a jail sentence than a well-deserved break in the action. My experience when people take disability leave is that it takes thirty days to really start their leave. The first thirty days is spent struggling with the uneasiness of not being frantically busy and overextended. Then there are the inevitable loose ends to tie up before they can really relax. It is only after the first thirty days that most people begin to spontaneously take really deep breaths.

Whitney also echoes the attitudes of many people who feel that taking the weekend off is a big deal or a special occasion. We all need regular timeouts. Sometimes scheduling your weekend timeouts on your calendar is helpful. When your time is booked on your calendar for relaxation, you may not be as tempted to allow work to take over.

Like many driven people, Whitney devoted her life to pleasing others. When you try to please everyone, everyone may love you, but you pay with your own life—and that is what was happening to Whitney. "It was not easy for me to say no," Whitney said. "I went into therapy because I realized that it was so hard for me to say no. One of the things my therapist had me do for three weeks was to just say no to everything that I was asked to do. After I was hospitalized, I understood where I was headed, and I knew that I couldn't keep living that kind of a lifestyle as I grew older and not end up with a major health crisis. So I started saying no." One of Whitney's successful techniques was to say to those asking for help, *Let me think about that before I answer.* Instead of immediately reacting, which is what Whitney had always done, by allowing herself time to think over a decision, she allowed herself to feel and to become aware of what she really did or did not *want* to do.

Doing unto YourSELF As You Would Do unto Others

What Whitney and millions of others need to understand is that there are beliefs and behaviors that served you when you were growing up that do not serve you at twenty, thirty, forty, fifty, sixty, and beyond. I once heard someone say, "If you keep doing what you're doing, you're going to keep getting what you are getting." This is your chance to make some decisions that will make your life what you want it to be. If you are suffering from or nearing burnout, it is not the time to say yes to anyone but yourSELF. This is the time to become SELFish.

Guidelines for listening to yourSELF
instead of everyone else

- Take a few deep, slow breaths, breathing in through your nose and out through your mouth.

- Remember your dreams. Are your dreams anxious, happy, chaotic? How do you feel when you awaken from a dream? Are your dreams trying to tell you something?

- Feel your feelings. Feel where they are in your body. Feel the places in your body where you feel tight, awkward, uncomfortable, and in pain. Yoga or stretching classes can help here.

- If possible, take some time every day to write about your thoughts, feelings, wishes, and dreams.

- Now that you have recognized what you are thinking and feeling and where you are hurting, first list and then reevaluate your priorities. Are you sure you want to run your life with the same outcomes, or would you rather discover new possibilities and choices?

- Consider finding someone who can help you hear yourself—a friend or a therapist. You would certainly ask for help for your child, computer, or car. Now is time to get help for yourSELF.

Guidelines for Doing for YourSELF Instead of for Everyone Else

Your needs are as important as everyone else's. Your needs are summarized in the Ten Simple Solutions.

> Simple Solution 1: Eat, Eat, Eat, All Day Long
> Simple Solution 2: Exercise Less
> Simple Solution 3: Calm Your Central Nervous System
> Simple Solution 4: Pay Off Your Sleep Debt
> Simple Solution 5: Let Go of Your Favorite Poison
> Simple Solution 6: Supplement a Tired Food Chain
> Simple Solution 7: Oxygenate Your Body
> Simple Solution 8: Learn About Hidden Toxins
> Simple Solution 9: Have Fun Every Day
> Simple Solution 10: Cultivate SELF-fulfillment

You cannot begin to incorporate these solutions into your life until you make yourSELF important enough. Everyone needs to devote time to themselves. If you do not take care of yourself you do not have time for meals, and you end up eating too much processed, junk, or fake foods. It takes time and attention to quit habits such as nicotine and caffeine, and if you do not devote time to yourself, you cannot accomplish these important goals. People who put others first often do not make enough time for rest and for sleep. Nor do they make time for calming activities, fun, play, and exercise.

You help everyone else. It is okay to ask for help for yourSELF. Do not be shy about talking with a good friend, a clergyman, or a therapist about reprioritizing your life.

Conquering Your Shoulds

Our early conditioning in life not only creates our psychogenes but also creates a list of shoulds. Our shoulds rigidly direct our behaviors.

For example, if your family were clean freaks, a little disorder in your house will arouse your psychogene. You believe that keeping your house spotless is a way of being successful, and your fear that your messiness means you are inferior → leads to anxiety about your failings → now your shoulds kick in like a nagging parent telling you that cleaning up your house will relieve your anxiety.

If your family prizes academic achievements, a B report card may arouse your pychogene. You believe that getting good grades is the way to be valued in life, and your fear of academic underachievement → leads to a sense of humiliation and failure over your B report card → your shoulds badger you into studying harder and harder, even all night.

If you grew up with a family who valued and praised football as manly, and you take up golf, you may arouse your psychogene. You believe that manly sports make a man superior, and your fear of not being manly → leads to a sense of shame and wimpiness that you took up golf → your shoulds never let you forget how you let your father down, and you may end up giving up golf and pursuing a more aggressive sport.

David Morrow, a forty-eight-year-old businessman, writer, and lecturer, has worked ten-, fifteen-, and even twenty-hour days for the last twenty years as a result of his shoulds. "I feel that I should be striving to be out there at the very top of my field, that I should be able to be accessible to people so that I can answer their questions. I also feel that I should be making a very good living for my family. I feel that I am responsible for keeping my home in good order. There are a lot of shoulds in my life. In fact, they go beyond shoulds. They are musts. There are lots of musts in my life, and I generally feel like I am failing at least part of them. So I really don't feel that there is any flexibility in my life. It was wearing because I never woke up in the morning without feeling that I was behind, and I had a tremendous amount to do that day just to try to pull even with the day. I almost never got to a point, even after thirteen hours of work, where I felt like I had a really productive day."

David believed that working harder than anyone else guaranteed safety, and his fear of negativity, tirades, and harsh criticism → led to apprehension that he was not doing enough → his shoulds led him to workaholic behavior → led to depression. Had David not recognized his psychogene and his shoulds and altered his behavior, he could have ended up working himself into a heart attack or stroke.

Forty-eight-year-old Vijay Mehta, who is juggling three full-time careers as tenured university professor, international consultant, and Internet entrepreneur, commented, "I am still a product of my Hindu upbringing. I was brought up with a strong sense of obligation, so it is very difficult for me to say no. So if you are constantly saying yes you find that you are always overcommitted and you are always being pulled in many different directions. I get a lot of my sense of worth and feeling useful from the activities that I engage in. It is part of my upbringing that you do things out of a sense of duty. You always put your duty first, even if it means self-sacrifice. Things like fun and pleasure are at the lowest rung in terms of priorities. Giving up on an obligation to just go out and have fun is very alien to the way that I was brought up."

Vijay's psychogene was that duty was his obligation and would bring a sense of self-worth, and his fear of not being dutiful enough

→ led to anxiety that he might not be sacrificing enough → his shoulds dogged him to the highest level of self-sacrifice → led to panic attacks.

Living up to Others' Expectations of You
Will Lead to Burnout

Thirty-five-year-old Conrad Lewis has always been what he calls a "high-fever" person. At six-foot-two and one hundred and-ninety-five pounds, with shoulder-length blond hair, Conrad radiates presence. He is articulate and thoughtful. "I always had this sense of destiny," he said. "I thought I was going to be a significant player in geopolitics. I planned to practice law in Latin America and work with multinationals and then go into the State Department and become secretary of state. I finished my undergraduate work in three years with two majors and graduated Phi Beta Kappa. Then I went to Georgetown University and I got a masters in Foreign Service, with a specialization in international business diplomacy. I came down with mononucleosis, which took me out of the loop for about a month. During that month I was involved in a near-fatal bicycling accident and spent six months recuperating."

If the time is right for you, an accident, an illness, an emotional breakdown, or the loss of a loved one can help you stop and pay attention to the things in life that are really important. Conrad was hit with illness and a life-threatening accident, but the time was not right for him to reevaluate his path. "As soon as I was well, I completed my class requirements for a double major, my master's thesis, and my exams in one year. I went right into Columbia Law School at twenty-one."

In the first year of law school, Conrad understood why Columbia has the highest suicide rate of first-year students of all of the law schools in the country. The demands were over and above what he had expected. Poised to command a six-figure salary after graduation, in his first year he was already being courted by some of the best law firms. "They would fly me to wherever their offices were and take me out to dinner in limousines." The heavy burden of expectations that he would be a brilliant lawyer forced Conrad to frantically study at all hours. He took up drinking coffee until he had "the worst intestinal discomfort of my life."

By the time first semester exams rolled around, twenty-two-year-old Conrad was distraught with anxiety and fear. "I was so crazed that in the middle of my exams I snapped. I went down the multiple choice questions just bubbling in whatever letter that I was inspired to bubble in. It was crazy behavior." Conrad barely passed one test and failed the other. "I lost it. I went on a drinking binge and went into a clinical depression. I managed to finish out my first year with reasonable grades. I went down to South Florida that summer and worked at a law firm. But I started to lose it again. I had suicidal thoughts. I was drinking like an animal and acting really badly. Three or four weekends during that summer I did cocaine for two days nonstop. I lost the opportunity to work with that law firm after graduation."

Conrad buckled emotionally on the first day in his first class of his second year of law school. He took a leave of absence then. To get his mind off his problems, he began practicing bodybuilding and yoga. He also unwittingly began following his body's natural rhythm by resting during the prime adrenal repair time. "I had this ritual of lying down in the afternoon at three o'clock for twenty-five minutes focusing on my breath going in and out and watching the images that would come up in my mind's eye. I would focus on that and empty my mind. I didn't call it meditation or even realize that was what I was doing." Conrad was not coached to rest in the afternoon. Because he listened to his body, he knew what to do.

Conrad began to track how many days he felt depressed a month and how many days he felt good. "As time went on, I saw that I would have ten days depressed where I stayed in bed all day and five days out of bed. Eventually two or three weeks would go by and I would only spend a couple of days depressed in bed. One day I was sitting at a red light and I realized I couldn't remember the last time that I had had a down day. I made a fist and I started yelling *yes, yes, yes.* I had finally healed myself from the darkest time in my life." Conrad healed himself by releasing himself from the grip of his shoulds, by respecting his own needs and wants, and by listening to his own body.

Before the end of Conrad's two-year leave of absence he knew he would not return to law school. Conrad's father, a Cuban man who struggled with lifelong alcohol and drug addictions, had immigrated to the United States in 1959 and had unrealized dreams of becoming a lawyer. Conrad now understands that he never really wanted a career in law to be his destiny. "I was just trying to please my dad who wanted to be a lawyer when he was younger but didn't manage to do it because of the Cuban Revolution."

Conrad believed that fulfilling his father's dream was his destiny, and his fear of not living up to his father's expectations → led to panic → his shoulds jumped right in and kept him in a near–death march toward "a brilliant law career." Fortunately, Conrad recognized his psychogene and conquered his shoulds.

Twenty-five-year-old Jason Wilkes, who is a dot com sales rep earning six figures, understands that he has long worked for his father's approval. "I attended Andover prep school outside Boston," Jason said. "It was highly competitive and I studied off the scale, often staying up all night. I had to prove to my dad that I was a quality kid. I learned early on that good grades got his attention and made him proud of me." Jason's aspirations are to "kick major butt in business and be successful like my uncles and my father."

Jason's psychogene is that being competitive and highly successful is a way to get his father's approval, and his fear that he can never achieve enough success to do so → led to landing a truly prestigious lucrative position → will Jason's shoulds follow him his entire life and continually tell him he is not successful enough? It remains to be seen. Only Jason can recognize his pychogene and his shoulds and, in his own words, kick them in the butt.

For the most part, people's shoulds are unconscious. They do not realize that the voice inside the head that directs them is not really their voice of choice. The voice of shoulds was implanted long before they were making many choices. In my opinion, Freud was right that we make most of our key decisions about life before we are five, but I also believe that he was wrong when he said there is nothing much you can do about it. In my clinical experience I have seen many people conquer their shoulds and learn how to make their own healthy choices. Like David, these people become aware of the inner dialogues and decisions that have been running their lives.

When I was a kid I used to recite: "Good, better, best, never let it rest, till the good is better and better is best." This poem may seem harmless, but it is this type of insidious programming that forms our shoulds. Years ago I discovered an awareness tool that I feel has saved my life and helped me and many of my patients to see more clearly through the inner fog. This exercise is a way to fully bring yourself into the present and become aware. This awareness will enable you to take charge instead of being bullied by unconscious directives from your past.

Write your shoulds in a notebook in one column, and in the opposite column list what you really want. I have personally written pages and pages of shoulds so that I could understand what was running my life. This practice helped me to learn to pay attention and to see my choices more clearly. When you recognize your shoulds, you can then pay attention, make new choices, and intercept many bad decisions.

Shoulds	What I Really Want
I should stay up all night cleaning my house so I have a perfectly clean house.	Although I want a clean house, what I really want is to sleep tonight.
I should have all the meals ready all the time for my family.	I want someone to cook for me once in awhile.
I should work hard to make a good living for my family.	I want to earn enough for my family to live well and for me to enjoy most weekends.

What are your shoulds?

_____

_____

_____

_____

Close your eyes and feel the feeling that you get in your neck or your belly when you think you should. It is not usually a good feeling. You might notice that you feel tight, drained, resistant, or resentful. Your thoughts have power. If you think *I should stay up all night cleaning so my house is perfectly clean,* you will probably get lost in your internal feelings of panic and dread. Instead of getting stuck with the awful thoughts and allowing those thoughts to reverberate in your biochemistry, stop, take some deep breaths, and collect yourself. Now you can respond in a new, healthy way. Instead of giving in to the panic, an alternative would be to do things differently. For example, if you feel that you should clean your house, once in a while accept and enjoy your house as "lived-in" and shift your focus to the warmth and comfort of your family as you get a good night's rest. When you allow yourSELF to respect your wants instead of your shoulds, you will actually become happier and more productive.

What are your wants?

_____

_____

_____

_____

The Beast of Never Enough

In the first ten to fifteen years of life, our parents teach us who we should be. Most of us swallow this programming and, without ever realizing it, carry it into adulthood. It usually takes an earthshaking event for people to see that they have other choices, that they can decide who they really are and who they want to become.

Conrad's shoulds nearly destroyed him. Compounding this problem, Conrad was infected with the inner beast of never enough. "My former aspirations came from wanting to appeal to that common vision of success that we have painted in America," Conrad said. "I know now that my problems in law school came from feelings of not being enough and not having enough."

My practice is filled with people who have enough wealth to buy anything they ever wanted. I have asked myself for years, how could it be that these people are not happy? The simple truth is that most people are not any happier because they have a lot of money or a lot of power.

Obviously the subject of happiness and wealth reaches far beyond the scope of this book. It is *not* my intention to tell you what you *should* do to be happy. This is an opportunity for *you* to decide if what you are doing now is the best choice for your life. What you do to change your relationship with your inner beast of never enough may be different from what the next person would do. The goal is not all or nothing. You do not have to entirely give up on your ambitions, but this is a chance to stop paying with your life for the accomplishment of your goals. The objective is to have reasonable goals and health in the same equation. Learning to care about yourself and valuing your own life is a powerful healing force, even if it feels strange to you at first.

Conrad is now married and is the father of three adorable little girls. He teaches Iyengar yoga, which is an extremely precise form of yoga, a practice that marries the mind and body. "I am in a constant state of deprogramming from when I was a little kid," Conrad commented. "One of the things that we learn in yoga is not to try and figure out 'why' but to do what is appropriate to do. In other words, if I get into a depression, I don't need to know why. Instead I need to do the things that I know will help me to get out of my depression, like eating the right foods, getting out in nature, and breathing."

Conrad has grown more confident in his ability to deal with adversity because he feels comfortable in his life. A significant factor in making changes in your life is to learn to have confidence in yourself. Our thoughts, for better or worse, create our neurotransmitters. Those neurotransmitters eventually make up who we are and how we feel. The exercises that follow can help you change negative thinking to create healthier neurotransmitters.

Creating Positive Thought Patterns and Healthy Neurotransmitters

Imagine that you have just gotten into a fender bender and it is your fault. Your adrenals react by immediately releasing adrenaline. Your heart begins to race; you feel like you are burning up; you are shaking. Your brain has sent an instant alert to your adrenals, and they are pumping adrenaline like crazy. All the adrenaline in your system is hyping you up and exacerbating your tendency to think negative thoughts at this moment. *What an idiot I am. This is going to cost a lot of money. Uh-oh, here comes the guy I hit. He's going to be mad. He's going to sue me.*

These thoughts are not going to create healthy neurotransmitters, nor will they enable you to function well in the moment. By allowing your thoughts to generate panic, you are focusing on what could be the worst possible scenario and rejecting potentially hopeful, positive outcomes. Your brain already registered danger the instant the accident occurred. Your body is now flooded with adrenaline. But remember, the release of adrenaline is roughly proportional to the intensity of a situation. In other words, the amount and intervals in which adrenaline is secreted is determined by the degree of danger perceived by the brain. A major pileup on the highway will elicit a larger and longer adrenaline response than a minor fender-bender. Of course, your response has something to do with it. If you allow yourself to panic, your brain will continue sending red alerts to your adrenals, which will continue to pump out adrenaline. And you will continue to feel like a quivering bowl of Jell-O.

When you do not allow yourself to panic and you purposefully calm yourself down, your brain will send a signal to your adrenals that the time of danger has passed or that the amount of adrenaline secreted is sufficient to deal with the situation. Your adrenals will stop secreting adrenaline. You will then have much more clarity to deal with your situation.

- Begin breathing slowly, deeply, and fully, inhaling through your nose and exhaling through your nose, relaxing your jaw as you exhale.

- Notice your breath and allow it to slow and deepen.

- Continue breathing and feel your body's rhythm beginning to change.

- Now pay attention to what you are thinking, and continue breathing deeply and slowly.

- Neutralize your scary, negative thoughts with thoughts that are positive and realistic, such as: *I can handle this. No one got hurt. This will turn out okay.*

- Allow yourself to feel how you are changing your experience of the moment.

- Notice that you are now feeling safer, calmer, and clearer of mind.

By doing this exercise in a moment of small or large crisis, you begin to neutralize the acidity of your panic reaction and calm your nervous system. You are in control by using the power of thought.

Instead of going home from a minor accident with a raging headache, you might end up thinking *look how lucky I am that it was only a fender-bender.*

The next step is deal with the thoughts, beliefs, habits, and feelings that regularly interfere with feeling safe. First, identify what kicks you out of your safe zone and write those things down on a list. Some examples might be:

You are kicked out of your safe zone when

- Your mother, father, or anyone else criticizes you

- You feel in a dependent position, such as answering to a boss

- A business deal that you have invested in shows signs of going south

- You open up your bank statement or credit card bill and it contains bad news

- You plan a party and people cancel at the last minute

- You get negative feedback from a superior at work

- You try on a piece of clothing and it is too tight

- You make a mistake, even if it was an accident

- Your mistakes, no matter how slight, are pointed out to you

- Someone laughs and you feel they are laughing at you

- You are in a dilemma and you do not know the answer

- You are in a situation in which you feel that you are not in control

What kicks you out of your safe zone?

_____

_____

_____

_____

When you keep a journal you can track day to day how your thoughts, beliefs, habits, and feelings can sabotage your ability to deal with life's big and small challenges. Begin to recognize how often you are your own worst critic/enemy and that you do not have to be so hard on yourself. You can then begin to change some of the things that you do and feel so that you are not always feeling threatened, anxious, and stressed. Remember that even a few changes can result in real progress.

Honoring Your Personal Rhythm

Each individual has a preferred way of working and living—a personal rhythm that is tied to his or her true wants and body desires. Some people love getting up at dawn—it just feels natural. Some people love cool weather; others thrive in warm weather. Some like going to bed at sunset; others love staying up half the night and sleeping until noon. Some like eating raw foods, others prefer cooked foods. If you thrive on being in nature, you would wither if you were forced to sit in an office and work on a computer. You would probably thrive as a naturalist or a forest ranger. Another person who loves computers and technology might enjoy working in an office but would shrivel in the hot sun. Part of the reason for the like or dislike of a pursuit is because it either fits or does not fit with your personal rhythm. Occupations all have a certain rhythm, tempo, and pace.

Illness often results from years of forcing your body to do what it does not want to do and from ignoring your true wants and needs. By not living your life according to your inherent rhythm, you are placing yourself under added stress. Anything that adds stress to your life will add stress to your adrenals. When your adrenals become depleted, your immune system is weakened and you are vulnerable to chronic conditions and illnesses.

Work and life decisions come with their own price tag. When you are chronically sick, a crucial question to ask yourself is "Am I going against my rhythm?" Being sick is often the only chance that people have to stop, look around, and see of the truth of their life. Why wait until you're sick? Now is the perfect time to take notice of what fits with your rhythm and what does not.

There are many complicated reasons that keep people stuck in life. While the logical solution would be to stop doing what makes you unhappy, obviously most do not have the freedom to change everything at once. In unguarded moments you may dream about quitting your job, moving to another place, or even changing your family situation. While those kinds of changes may seem like the solution, it may be that all you need to do to get unstuck in life is to take deep breaths, eat balanced meals, get a little more exercise, and sleep more soundly. It is truly amazing how different life can look when you feel better.

If you are on the path to burnout or if you have reached Burned Out and you find that adhering to the other simple solutions for at least eight weeks has not gotten you out of your rut, now is a good time to look further. If you are really honest with yourself, you might realize that you no longer want to force your body to do what it does not want to do. You could be in the wrong career, living in the wrong place, with the wrong person. Only you can make the decision to make a change. You are the only one who can say "This isn't working."

Conrad was pressed into law school by his inner expectations. Although he is a brilliant man, law school was not right for him. He was not respecting his personal wants and needs. After years of forcing himself to go against his rhythm, he crashed. When he discovered and followed his rhythm and did what he really wanted and needed to do, he found health and happiness. If it is at all possible for you to make changes, there is no time like the present. Begin considering how you can alter your life to better fit with your personal rhythm. I am sure you will be rewarded in ways beyond your expectations. I see it happen regularly.

What are your true desires for your life?
What really matters to you?

_____

_____

_____

_____

If you feel that you are living a life that does not suit your personal rhythm, be honest with yourself. Even if it is impossible to change your life right now, at least acknowledge your true desires and needs. This will be your first step in finding ways to create more of the life you have always wanted and deserved.

Paying Attention Instead of Paying Dues

Changing your life to better fit with your wants and needs starts with paying attention to what is really going on inside you. Most of us do not pay much attention to ourSELVES and how we are running our lives. We rarely even recognize who is truly running our lives. Too often we become numb to much of the inner dialogue we have, yet our inner dialogue is running the majority of our decisions and reactions. I find it amazing how much garbage passes through my mind every day. Sometimes as I listen and ask myself, "Who said that?" or "Where did that come from?" When thoughts come out of my mouth that I did not mean to say, I am clear now that it is because I was not paying attention to what was going on in my mind.

Paying attention is free, paying dues is expensive. When you pay attention you can avoid paying dues. The meter maid and the traffic cop thrive on your not paying attention to traffic laws. When you do not pay attention to your body and your needs, you end up paying dues. When you continually abuse your body or deny your true wants and needs, the chances of knowing and reaching your goals are slim. These are costly dues. You do not need to pay with your life. When you pay attention to nourishing your body, appreciating yourSELF, and treating yourSELF with respect, you will be healthier and have more energy and attention to fuel your path to success.

Guidelines for paying attention

- Breathe deeply throughout this exercise.

- Listen to your thoughts and the chatter in your mind. When you really pay attention, what do you hear?

- Take a few moments to notice where you are in your day and in your life.

- Instead of thinking of what you are going to do next, stay with thinking about the present and where you are right at this moment.

- Notice tension in your body, and let that lead you to uncover your unconscious thoughts and desires.

- Breathe even more deeply and slowly now.

- Ask yourself honestly if there are ways in which you can be better to yourSELF.

- Breathe deeply and visualize the Simple Solutions you can begin to include in your life and how much better you will feel.

Now that you have experienced this moment of clarity, practice bringing yourself back into this experience as often as you can. Soon you will begin to notice a welcome calmness in your body and mind. The Olympic and competitive athletes who visualize their successful outcomes in advance are the ones who win the gold.

Changing Your Psychogene Equation

Now that you have the tools to make simple yet powerful changes in your life, it will be easier for you to see how you can change your psychogene equation. Earlier in this book we reviewed unhealthy psychogene equations. Here they are again, revised to show how they can become healthy equations.

Variations on the revised healthy psychogene equation

Your belief that you are adequate and that you can succeed → leads to self confidence → leads to working reasonable hours and getting enough sleep → leads to success, good health, vitality, and normal body weight.

Your belief that it is okay to let your guard down occasionally and admit that you are human → leads to a sense of humility that people respect → leads to a balanced work and personal lifestyle → leads to success, good health, vitality, and normal body weight.

Your belief that everyone has a different body type and your satisfaction with yours → leads to self-respect → leads to eating a balanced diet of real, whole foods → leads to success, good health, vitality, and normal body weight.

Your belief that your worth does not hinge on success, power, money, and status but is measured in deeper, more personal, spiritual terms → leads to the knowledge that your spiritual quest is a lifelong pursuit → leads to better overall balance in your work and personal life → leads to success, good health, vitality, and normal body weight.

Your belief that you are an intelligent person → leads to confidence about facing life's challenges → leads to accepting and moving past your mistakes → leads to success, good health, vitality, and normal body weight.

Your belief that it is acceptable to show your emotions at times → leads to a sense of relief that you do not have to try to solve everyone else's problems → leads to saying no when people ask things of you that you do not want to do → leads to success, good health, vitality, and normal body weight.

Your belief that although you may be the sole breadwinner of your family, you are made of flesh and bones and can only do so much → leads to a sense of camaraderie and teamwork within your family that brings you closer together → leads to working reasonable hours and being there when your family needs you → leads to success, good health, vitality, and normal body weight.

What is your new healthy psychogene equation?

_____→ led to

What is your new psychogene—your beliefs and strengths?

_____→ led to

What positive emotion can you attach to your new psychogene?

_____→ led to

What new behaviors have you developed as a result of
that positive emotion?

_____

What positive emotional and/or physical results have you
enjoyed?

Develop a Sense of Purpose and Meaning in Your Life

Without a purpose, the pressures and pain of life can lead a person to
give up hope. It helps to have a sense of meaning in your life. You can
better rise above what life throws at you and know that your own life
has a purpose and that you are important. David Morrow said, "I see
my life as being an effort to learn as much as I can to help other
people live better lives. In the process I am trying to develop habits so
that I can also enjoy a few of life's pleasures and take good care of my
health." Songwriter Grace Wolczak strives to develop and nourish a
sense of meaning through her work. "I thank God daily for giving me
guidance and enriching me with new opportunities."

Life is often difficult, sometimes even unfair or cruel. I am not
suggesting that you pretend that your life is not at times difficult or
painful. At the same time, life's problems do not need to lead us to
feeling hopeless.

When many people think of the meaning of life, they immediately assume they must pursue a life of total self-sacrifice. This is not
true. I have learned from experience that when people take care of

What gives you a sense of meaning in life?

_____

_____

_____

_____

themselves, their sense of meaning in life _increases_. When you take care of yourSELF you will avoid burnout, and there will be so much more of YOU to give.

Simple Solution 10: Cultivate SELF-fulfillment Tailored to your stage of burnout

Driven and Dragging

____ Even though you feel invincible, you cannot take on the world indefinitely. Learn to say no to at least some of the requests people make of you.

____ At these stages, if you listen to yourSELF instead of everyone else, you will make healthier choices for your life.

____ It is easy in the Driven and Dragging stages to be dictated to by your SHOULDS. Begin weeding them out now.

____ If you live your life according to others' expectations of you, will you be happy?

____ Cowering at the demands of your inner beast of never enough will perpetuate lifelong servitude. Why not slay that beast as soon as possible?

____ Learn to recognize and begin to change what kicks you out of your safe zone. Your life will be happier.

____ You can change your psychogene equation now and live a healthier life.

____ Developing a sense of meaning in your life will carry you through.

Losing It

___ If you have not learned to say no to people's requests of you, chances are you have been run ragged by their demands. Practice saying no now.

___ It is not too late to learn how to listen to yourSELF instead of everyone else. Ask yourself: What do I really want?

___ Begin learning how to take care of yourSELF instead of constantly tending to everyone else's needs. This includes family, co-workers and even your boss.

___ Has your life been run by your SHOULDS? Recognize now where your SHOULDS have brought you and begin to deal with them.

___ If you have been living up to others' expectations of you, you know now that it brings unhappiness. Decide what makes you happy and follow that path.

___ Face off with your beast of never enough now before you slide any further into burnout.

___ What kicks you out of your safe zone? Do you really want to be ruled by those emotions? Deal with these issues and get on with your life.

___ You have true desires and dreams for your life. This is a great time to ask yourself what really matters to you.

___ Midway to burnout and still ruled by your psychogene equation? Only you can change that.

___ Why wait until your life feels meaningless? Develop a sense of meaning in your life now.

Hitting the Wall and Burned Out

___ If you are Hitting the Wall, saying yes to people's requests of you is a factor in your adrenal fatigue. Say no, to save your life. If you are burned out, only the most insensitive person would ask you to do something for them. But those people do exist. Say no to everyone but yourSELF.

___ While you are healing, listen to yourSELF instead of every-one else. You know what you need to do.

___ There is no room in your life for SHOULDS now. Conquer them now so you can live the rest of your life in peace.

___ Others will still have expectations of you, no matter how fa-tigued or ill you are. Recognize that you are the only person who can choose to accept or reject those expectations.

___ Funny how your beast of never enough can survive any-thing. You may be hitting the wall, or burned out, but the beast is alive and kicking. This is a great time to deal with your beast once and for all.

___ There is nothing like fatigue, burnout, and illness to kick even the most stalwart person out of his of her safe zone. Take this healing time to recognize and begin to change what kicks you out of your safe zone. And deal with it.

___ Reflect now on your true desires for your life. What really matters to you? You can make those changes now.

___ You can see now where your psychogene equation has led you. This is truly a now-or-never opportunity to change that equation forever.

___ It takes courage to overcome extreme adrenal fatigue and burnout, but you can do it. Developing or renewing a sense of meaning in your life will speed your recovery.

Part Three

Eat Regular Balanced
Meals of Real Whole Food
to Take Back Your Life

Fourteen-Day
Meal Plans
and Recipes

*An easy guide to help you
change your eating habits,
one step at a time*

There are some simple things you can do to begin
to change your eating habits. I suggest making
small changes. If you are in Losing It, Hitting the Wall, or Burned Out,
your adrenals will need more support. Do what you can without making yourself more stressed out.

A two-week meal plan follows for nourishing your tired adrenals,
regaining your health, and dropping those few extra pounds. These
meals are alkalinizing and low carbohydrate—about 15 grams per
meal and 10 grams or less per snack. *If you need more carbohydrates, increase your intake based on the carbohydrate guidelines in chapter 4.* Bread is
a processed food and high in carbohydrate. If you eat bread, buy
freshly made bakery bread or low-carbohydrate bread.

The recipes for these meals begin on page 317, immediately after
the plan. Power Drink recipes begin on page 334.

14-Day Adrenal Support Meal Plan

Day 1

PRE-BREAKFAST (optional): Protein power drink.

BREAKFAST: Santa Barbara Scrambled Eggs. Sliced tomatoes. One slice buttered low-carbohydrate whole grain toast. Hot herbal tea.

SNACK: Two stalks celery with ⅓ cup hummus. Iced herbal tea.

LUNCH: Tuna Salad (see recipe on page 320). Tropical fruit salad made with a total of ¾ cup mixed papaya, mango, and kiwi topped with unsweetened whipped cream or sweetened with a small amount of stevia. Iced herbal tea with lemon slices.

SNACK: ¼ cup sunflower seeds.

DINNER: Grilled pork chop. One-half baked potato with butter, sour cream, and chives. Salad of organic greens, carrots, tomatoes, and cucumbers with Walnut Dressing.

GRANDMOTHER'S SNACK FOR INSOMNIACS: ½ cup warmed raw milk. One fresh fig.

Day 2

PRE-BREAKFAST (optional): Protein power drink.

BREAKFAST: ½ cup cottage cheese with ½ cup watermelon.

SNACK: ¼ cup Dr. Hanley's Alkalinizing Trail mix.

LUNCH: Take-out or homemade chicken or tofu Caesar salad made with Romaine lettuce and anchovies, topped with grilled chicken and Caesar salad dressing or Creamy Vinaigrette. Iced herbal tea. ½ cup berries.

DINNER: All-Day Beef Stew—limit carrots and potatoes to a total of ½ cup. Cucumber salad with Creamy Cucumber Marinade.

Grandmother's snack for insomniacs: String cheese with ¼ banana.

Day 3

Pre-breakfast (optional): Protein power drink.

Breakfast: ¼ cup Nancy Deville's Breakfast Muesli. Hard-boiled eggs. Hot herbal tea.

Snack: Two Ak Mak crackers—or any other cracker made without hydrogenated fats—with 2 tablespoons almond butter.

Lunch: Ham and cheese melt made with nitrate-free Black Forest ham and your choice cheese on one slice buttered low-carbohydrate whole grain bread. Vegetable soup—from your health food store deli.

Snack: ¼ cup pumpkin seeds.

Dinner: Chicken with Sweet and Sour Sauce. ⅓ cup brown rice. Salad of sliced cucumbers, tomatoes, chopped fresh dill, and Cucumber Marinade.

Grandmother's snack for insomniacs: String cheese. ½ apple.

Day 4

Pre-breakfast (optional): Protein power drink.

Breakfast: Nitrate-free turkey sausages. Scrambled eggs. One piece buttered whole grain low-carbohydrate toast. Hot herbal tea.

Snack: Chicken Liver Paté—see recipe, or buy it at your health food store deli—on 2 Finn Crisp crackers, or any other cracker made without hydrogenated fats.

Lunch: Crab Salad. Asparagus Soup. Small bunch grapes. Iced herbal tea.

Snack: One-half medium orange with 3 ounces grilled tofu—from your health food store deli. Or protein power drink.

Dinner: Mama's Meat Loaf. ⅓ cup mashed potatoes with butter. Steamed broccoli. Mixed green salad with cucumbers, tomatoes, bell peppers, onions, and Dr. Hanley's Alkalinizing Buttermilk dressing. Iced herbal tea.

Grandmother's snack for insomniacs: Cottage cheese rolled into thinly sliced turkey breast.

Day 5

Pre-breakfast (optional): Protein power drink.

Breakfast: Classic Egg Salad. One piece buttered whole grain low-carbohydrate toast. Sliced cucumbers. Iced herbal tea.

Snack: 1 rice cake mounded with ½ cup cottage cheese and a slice of avocado. Or protein power drink.

Lunch: Turkey cheeseburger with tomatoes and grilled onions on one half whole grain bun, drenched in Creamy Vinaigrette. Iced herbal tea.

Snack: ½ apple and 6 almonds.

Dinner: Lamb chops. ¼ cup applesauce. Steamed green beans. Mixed greens salad with Creamy Vinaigrette. 1 ounce fruit juice mixed in 10 to 12 ounces sparkling water.

Grandmother's snack for insomniacs: Sliced turkey roll-ups. One fresh fig.

Day 6

Pre-breakfast (optional): Protein power drink.

Breakfast: ½ cup cooked rolled oats with butter and ¼ cup coconut milk. Two soft-boiled eggs. Hot herbal tea.

SNACK: Two Ak Mak crackers—or any other cracker made without hydrogenated fats—topped with 2 tablespoons cream cheese and smoked salmon.

LUNCH: Grilled nitrate-free chicken sausages with Dijon mustard. ½ cup baked yams with butter. California Coleslaw with California Coleslaw Dressing. Iced herbal tea.

SNACK: One-half apple with 2 tablespoons aflatoxin-free peanut butter. Or protein power drink.

DINNER: Halibut marinated in Cilantro Pesto and baked. Two small potatoes basted with extra virgin olive oil, sprinkled with fresh rosemary, and baked. Steamed spinach with butter. Mixed greens salad with Basic Dressing. Iced herbal tea.

GRANDMOTHER'S SNACK FOR INSOMNIACS: Turkey and swiss cheese roll-up. 2 tablespoons raisins.

Day 7—Emergency Rescue Lounge Day Menu

PRE-BREAKFAST (optional): Protein power drink.

BREAKFAST: Breakfast sandwich made with scrambled eggs, sliced soy sausages, cheese of your choice, and sliced tomato on one slice buttered whole grain low-carbohydrate toast. Hot herbal tea.

SNACK: One rice cake topped with sliced cheese of your choice, avocado, and a drizzle of Dr. Hanley's Alkalinizing Buttermilk Dressing.

LUNCH: Nancy Deville's Emergency Rescue Lounge Day Chicken Soup. 3 wheat melba toasts, or any other cracker made without hydrogenated fat. Iced herbal tea.

SNACK: ⅛ cup walnuts and ½ cup berries with unsweetened whipped cream or sweetened with a small amount of stevia.

DINNER: High Enzyme Salad. Grilled turkey patties. Hot herbal tea—detox tea optional.

GRANDMOTHER'S SNACK FOR INSOMNIACS: ½ cup warmed raw milk. One-quarter apple with 1 tablespoon almond butter.

Day 8

PRE-BREAKFAST (optional): Protein power drink.

BREAKFAST: Breakfast steak with ⅓ cup hash-browned potatoes fried in butter or coconut butter. Sliced tomatoes. Hot herbal tea.

SNACK: Nancy Deville's Favorite Deviled Eggs. Carrot sticks. One-half apple.

LUNCH: One-half whole grain pita pocket with sliced roast beef, cheese slices, sprouts, tomatoes, and onions, with horseradish sauce. Iced herbal tea.

SNACK: 1 tablespoon cashew butter on one rice cake.

DINNER: Grilled Mahi Mahi and ⅓ cup brown rice smothered in Coconut Curry Sauce. Cucumber and red bell pepper salad with Creamy Cucumber Marinade. Iced herbal tea.

GRANDMOTHER'S SNACK FOR INSOMNIACS: Feta cheese rolled up in one-half corn tortilla.

Day 9

PRE-BREAKFAST (optional): Protein power drink.

BREAKFAST: 1 cup cottage cheese. ¼ cup cubed melon. Hot herbal tea.

SNACK: Classic Egg Salad on two Ak Mak Crackers—or any other cracker made without hydrogenated fats.

LUNCH: One to two sirloin patties. Beefsteak and mozzarella salad with Basil Pesto. ½ cup diced cantaloupe. 1 ounce fruit juice in 8 to 10 ounces sparkling water.

SNACK: Protein power drink.

DINNER: Baked Salmon. Steamed broccoli and ⅓ cup butternut squash with butter. Mixed green salad with Basic Dressing. 1 ounce fruit juice in 8 to 10 ounces sparkling water.

GRANDMOTHER'S SNACK FOR INSOMNIACS: ½ cup warm raw milk. One Finn Crisp with 1 tablespoon almond butter.

Day 10

PRE-BREAKFAST (optional): Protein power drink.

BREAKFAST: Scrambled eggs with turkey bacon. One slice buttered whole grain low-carbohydrate toast. Cucumber slices.

SNACK: ¼ cup Spicy Mixed Nuts.

LUNCH: Classic Chicken Salad. ¾ cup sliced strawberries with unsweetened whipped cream or sweetened with a small amount of stevia.

DINNER: Stir-fry made with tofu, snow peas, diced onion, broccoli, fresh ginger, sweet red pepper. ⅓ cup brown rice with butter. Mixed greens salad with salad greens, sprouts, shredded carrots, scallions, and cilantro with Basic Dressing.

GRANDMOTHER'S SNACK FOR INSOMNIACS: One Finn Crisp—or any other cracker made without hydrogenated fats with 1 tablespoon almond butter. ½ cup warmed raw milk.

Day 11

PRE-BREAKFAST (optional): Protein power drink.

BREAKFAST: Sirloin steak with ⅓ cup hash-browned potatoes fried in butter or coconut butter. Hot herbal tea.

SNACK: Nancy Deville's Favorite Deviled Eggs. Ten cherries.

LUNCH: Cottage Cheese and Chopped Vegetable Salad.

SNACK: Guacamole—homemade or from your health food store deli—with carrot and celery sticks. Or protein power drink.

DINNER: Grilled steak with Horseradish Sauce. One-half potato cut in wedges, dredged in extra virgin olive oil and fresh rosemary, and baked until crisp. Cucumber and tomato salad with Creamy Cucumber Marinade.

GRANDMOTHER'S SNACK FOR INSOMNIACS: ½ cup warmed raw milk. One-quarter apple with 1 tablespoon almond butter.

Day 12

PRE-BREAKFAST (optional): Protein power drink.

BREAKFAST: One piece of French toast made with cream and beaten egg and fried in butter or coconut butter—dusted with cinnamon for sweetness. Scrambled eggs. Hot herbal tea.

SNACK: Two fish-of-choice sushi rolls—from your health food store deli.

LUNCH: Cottage Cheese Salad with Chopped Vegetables. ¼ cup fresh pineapple. Iced herbal tea.

DINNER: Mediterranean Shrimp. ⅓ cup brown rice with butter. Green salad with Basic Dressing. Iced herbal tea.

GRANDMOTHER'S SNACK FOR INSOMNIACS: ½ cup whole plain yogurt (cow or goat) with one-quarter sliced banana.

Day 13—Detox Menu

PRE-BREAKFAST (optional): Protein power drink.

BREAKFAST: Spinach and mushroom omelet. Sliced tomatoes. One-half grapefruit. Detox tea.

SNACK: Beiler's Broth.

LUNCH: High Enzyme Salad. ⅓ cup hummus with carrot and bell pepper sticks.

SNACK: ¼ cup Dr. Hanley's Alkalinizing Trail Mix.

DINNER: Simple Lemon-Roasted Chicken. ½ cup turnips with butter—roast turnips with chicken. Salad of sliced bell peppers, onions, tomatoes, and cucumbers with Basic Dressing. 1 ounce fruit juice in 8 to 10 ounces sparkling water.

GRANDMOTHER'S SNACK FOR INSOMNIACS: ½ cup warmed raw milk. One-quarter apple with 1 tablespoon cashew butter.

Day 14—Emergency Rescue Lounge Day Menu

PRE-BREAKFAST (optional): Protein power drink.

BREAKFAST: Open-faced breakfast sandwich made with one piece of whole grain low-carbohydrate toast topped with 1 tablespoon cream cheese, 2 slices nitrate-free Black Forest ham, and two poached eggs. Hot herbal tea.

SNACK: ½ cup cottage cheese. One-half pear.

LUNCH: Nancy Deville's Alkalinizing Tomato Soup. Grilled nitrate-free turkey sausages. ¾ cup sliced blueberries with unsweetened whipped cream or sweetened with a small amount of stevia. Iced herbal tea with lemon slices.

SNACK: Protein power drink.

DINNER: Broiled sea bass with Cilantro Marinade. ⅓ cup wild rice with butter. California Coleslaw with dressing. Iced herbal tea.

GRANDMOTHER'S SNACK FOR INSOMNIACS: ½ cup whole plain yogurt. ⅛ cup walnuts.

Recipes

⌒

Throughout this book you have learned about the health hazards of eating processed, junk, and fake foods. These products affect how you feel—and they also affect how you look. If you care about how you feel and look, there is no substitute for preparing and eating real food. Your meals do not have to be complicated or gourmet—but they do have to be made out of real food. Since we have all gotten away from preparing meals, it takes a bit of practice to get back in the habit. Several chefs have contributed easy-to-make recipes to give you a well-rounded repertoire of balanced meals that you can make using real, whole foods.

You will find here recipes for egg dishes, breakfast grain dishes, salads, soups, meat, poultry, and fish dishes, dressings, marinades, and sauces, snacks, and power drinks.

Always use real, whole foods, such as whole cream cheese, cottage cheese, and yogurt. Be aware that low-fat or nonfat foods have the fat removed only to be replaced with gums and sugar. You are much better off using the real, whole product. Buy heavy cream, without added chemicals. Use pure-, cold-, or expeller-pressed oils, including pure pressed extra virgin olive oil and mayonnaise made from pure-, cold-, or expeller-pressed monounsaturated oil. Most important, eat organic foods whenever possible.

EGG DISHES

Santa Barbara Scrambled Eggs
from *The Schwarzbein Principle Vegetarian Cookbook*

4 eggs

2 tablespoons heavy cream

freshly ground black pepper, to taste

2 tablespoons unsalted butter

1 cup sliced brown or white mushrooms

3 ounces cream cheese, cut into ½ inch cubes

2 tablespoons grated Parmesan cheese

2 tablespoons slivered fresh basil, or 1 tablespoon dried basil

1 tablespoon minced fresh parsley

sea salt, to taste

• In a medium bowl, using a fork, whisk eggs, cream, and black pepper. Set aside.

• In a 10-inch nonstick skillet, melt butter over medium-high heat. When butter is hot and bubbly, add sliced mushrooms. Cook until mushrooms are softened, about 5 minutes. Drain excess liquids.

• Pour beaten egg mixture over mushrooms. Reduce heat to medium. Gently stir egg mixture with wooden spoon, about 1 minute, until eggs begin to set. Sprinkle cream cheese, Parmesan cheese, basil, and parsley evenly over eggs. Continue folding until cheese is melted and eggs are set. Serve immediately.

Makes 2 servings.

Classic Egg Salad
from *The Schwarzbein Principle Cookbook*

8 hard-boiled eggs

1 tablespoon Dijon mustard

½ cup mayonnaise

1 tablespoon capers, rinsed and drained (optional)

1 tablespoon minced fresh parsley

½ teaspoon dried dill

freshly ground black pepper, to taste

dash cayenne pepper

sea salt, to taste

• To hard-boil eggs, place eggs in a saucepan and cover with cold water. Bring to a boil uncovered. Allow to boil for 1 minute, then cover, remove from heat, and let sit undisturbed for 10 minutes. Rinse eggs under cold water. Crack shells, peel, and rinse eggs and chop fine.

• In a medium bowl combine chopped egg with remaining ingredients. Taste, and adjust seasonings.

Makes 4 servings.

Nancy Deville's Breakfast Muesli

½ cup rolled oats

⅛ cup slivered almonds or chopped walnuts

⅛ cup dried shredded unsweetened coconut

¼ teaspoon cinnamon, to taste

1½ cups raw milk

½ cup whole, plain yogurt

⅛ cup raisins

• Stir together and let soak in the refrigerator all night.

Makes 4 servings.

SALADS

Classic Chicken Salad
from *The Schwarzbein Principle Cookbook*

2 bay leaves

4 boneless, skinless chicken breasts

2 teaspoons minced fresh parsley

½ cup finely diced celery stalks

½ cup chopped raw pecans

⅔ cup mayonnaise

6 cups mixed salad greens

2 teaspoons Dijon mustard

1 teaspoon curry powder (optional)

sea salt, to taste

freshly ground black pepper, to taste

4 fresh parsley sprigs for garnish

Creamy Vinaigrette

• Bring 1 inch of water and bay leaves to a boil in a skillet. Reduce heat to medium. Add chicken, cover, and poach until cooked through, about 20 minutes, turning once. Do not overcook. Let cool and shred with fingers.

• In a large bowl, combine all ingredients except salad greens, vinaigrette, and parsley sprigs. Blend well with fork. Taste, and adjust seasonings.

• Line 4 individual plates with washed and dried salad greens. Mound greens with chicken salad and garnish with whole parsley sprigs. Pass Creamy Vinaigrette.

Makes 4 main-course servings.

Tuna or Crab Salad

from *The Schwarzbein Principle Cookbook*

13 ounces canned tuna or crab, drained and flaked

⅓ cup mayonnaise

2 teaspoons drained and rinsed capers

6 cups mixed salad greens

½ cup minced celery stalks

2 tablespoons minced red onion

¼ cup fresh lemon juice

1 tablespoon Dijon mustard

sea salt, to taste

freshly ground pepper, to taste

Creamy Vinaigrette

· In a medium bowl, using a fork, combine all ingredients, except salad greens and vinaigrette. Mix well.

· Line 4 individual plates with salad greens. Scoop tuna or crab salad over mixed greens. Spoon Creamy Vinaigrette over salad.

Makes 4 side-dish servings.

High Enzyme Salad

from *Nourishing Traditions*

1 cup sprouted sunflower seeds

4 carrots, peeled and grated

1 cucumber, peeled and finely chopped

1 red pepper, seeded and finely chopped

1 bunch green onions, finely chopped

2 ounces grated raw cheddar cheese (optional)

¾ cup Basic Dressing

1 avocado, sliced

radicchio or red lettuce leaves

· To sprout sunflower seeds, use hulled sunflower seeds purchased in airtight containers. Pour into a bowl and rinse. Rinse twice per day. Sprouts will be ready to eat in 12 to 18 hours. Mix sprouted sunflower seeds, carrots, cucumber, pepper, onions, and cheese with dressing. Serve on radicchio or lettuce leaves and garnish with avocado slices.

Makes 4 servings.

California Coleslaw

from *The Schwarzbein Principle Cookbook*

1½ cups shredded green cabbage

1½ cups shredded red cabbage

1 coarsely grated carrot

3 celery stalks, sliced thin diagonally

½ thinly sliced red onion (optional)

¼ cup minced parsley

California Coleslaw Dressing

· In a large bowl, toss all ingredients with California Cole Slaw Dressing. Refrigerate at least 1 hour before serving.

Makes 4 side-dish servings.

Cottage Cheese Salad with Chopped Vegetables

from *The Schwarzbein Principle Vegetarian Cookbook*

2 finely diced carrots

3 finely chopped scallions

1 finely chopped red bell pepper

3 finely chopped celery stalks

1 tablespoon minced fresh parsley

1 tablespoon minced fresh chives

2 cups whole cottage cheese

sea salt, to taste

freshly ground black pepper, to taste

4 cups mixed salad greens

· In a medium bowl, using a fork, mix all ingredients, except salad greens, with cottage cheese. Line 4 individual plates with mixed salad greens. Mound cottage cheese salad on top. Serve immediately.

Makes 4 side-dish servings.

SOUPS

Nancy Deville's Alkalinizing Tomato Soup

2 cups organic chicken or vegetable broth

12 large, vine-ripened organic tomatoes, coarsely chopped

8-ounce jar sun-dried tomatoes in extra virgin expeller-pressed olive oil

one large bunch fresh organic basil, stems, and flowers, coarsely chopped

sea salt, to taste

freshly ground black pepper, to taste

cayenne pepper, to taste

1 tablespoon freshly ground nutmeg, or ½ teaspoon store-bought

1 cup heavy cream

- In a large soup pot, over medium heat, cook tomatoes in chicken broth one-half hour or until tomatoes are mushy. Add basil and cook 1 to 2 minutes or until wilted. Remove from stove. **Cool completely before blending.** If soup is hot when blending, to prevent the hot soup from popping off the top of your blender, **blend 1 cup at a time.** Drape a dish towel over the top and hold **firmly** as you blend each batch. Rinse and wipe pot.

- Pour the blended soup back into the pot and season with cayenne pepper, nutmeg, and salt and pepper to taste. To serve, heat soup piping hot. Ladle into bowls and pour about 2 tablespoons cream into the center of each bowl.

Makes about 10 servings.

Nancy Deville's Emergency Rescue Lounge Day Chicken Soup

1 whole organic stewing chicken, about 4 pounds

4 quarts (equals four 32-ounce containers) organic chicken broth

3 carrots, coarsely chopped

4 celery stalks with leaves, coarsely chopped

1 bunch coarsely chopped fresh parsley

3 bay leaves

sea salt, to taste

- In a large soup pot, bring whole chicken and broth to a boil. You will not have any foam if the chicken is organic. Otherwise, skim off foam as it collects on the surface. When no more foam appears, add remaining ingredients, except finely sliced carrots and celery. Reduce heat to low and cook below a simmer, covered, for 6 to 8 hours.

- Remove soup from heat and cool. Strain broth. Discard vegetables, chicken skin, fat, and bones. Shred meat with your fingers and reserve. In the same pot, over medium heat, cook carrots and freshly ground black pepper, to taste

3 finely sliced carrots

2 finely sliced celery stalks

celery in broth until soft, about 10 minutes. Add shredded meat, heat to piping hot and serve.

Makes about 8 servings.

Asparagus Soup
from *Nourishing Traditions*

3 medium onions, peeled and chopped

3 tablespoons butter

1½ quarts chicken stock

4 red potatoes, washed and cut into quarters

2 bunches tender asparagus, with tough ends removed, cut into ¼ inch pieces

2 cloves garlic, peeled and coarsely chopped

sea salt and pepper

1 cup sour cream

• Sauté onions gently in butter until tender. Add stock, garlic, and potatoes. Bring to a boil and skim. Simmer for about 15 minutes. Add asparagus and simmer another 10 minutes or so until tender. Blend with a handheld blender. Pass the soup through a strainer to remove any strings from the asparagus. Season to taste. Reheat gently. Ladle into heated bowls and serve with a dollop of sour cream.

Makes 6 servings.

Bieler Broth

4 medium squash, such as zucchini, yellow, or summer, washed, ends removed, and sliced

1 pound string beans, ends and strings removed

2 stalks celery, chopped

2 bunches parsley, stems removed

fresh herbs such as thyme or tarragon, tied together with a string

1 quart water

• Health pioneer Henry Bieler, M.D., recommended this broth for cleansing and for overall health. This combination of vegetables is ideal for restoring acid-alkaline and sodium-potassium balance to organs and glands—especially the sodium-loving adrenal glands. Bieler broth is highly recommended for those under stress or suffering from stress-related conditions.

• In a large soup pot, bring all ingredients to a boil. Skim off any foam and simmer, uncovered, for 30 minutes. Remove herbs.

Makes 2 quarts.

MEAT, POULTRY, AND FISH

Mama's Meat Loaf

from *The Schwarzbein Principle Cookbook*

1 tablespoon olive oil

½ cup chopped onion

2 minced garlic cloves

2 pounds ground beef, pork, or turkey

2 eggs

½ cup fresh or dried whole grain bread crumbs

½ cup finely chopped fresh parsley

1 tablespoon dried oregano

1 tablespoon dried basil

sea salt, to taste

freshly ground black pepper, to taste

· Preheat oven to 350˚.

· In a medium nonstick skillet, heat oil over medium-high heat. When oil is hot, add onion and garlic and sauté until softened, about 5 minutes.

· In a large bowl, combine all ingredients and mix well, using your hands or a wooden spoon. Lightly oil a loaf pan or 9-inch pie pan. Shape the meat into the pan. Bake about 1½ hours.

Makes 6 servings.

All-Day Beef Stew

from *Nourishing Traditions*

3 pounds stew beef, cut into 1-inch pieces

1 cup red wine

3 to 4 cups beef stock

4 tomatoes, peeled, seeded, and chopped, or 1 can tomatoes

4 tablespoons tomato paste

6 whole cloves

½ teaspoon black peppercorns

several springs fresh thyme, tied together

2 cloves garlic, peeled and crushed

2 to 3 small red potatoes

1 pound carrots, peeled and cut into sticks

sea salt and pepper

· Marinate meat in red wine overnight. Place all ingredients except for potatoes and carrots in a flameproof casserole and cook gently in a 250° oven for about 12 hours. You may also use a crock pot set at medium temperature. Add carrots and potatoes during the last hour. Season to taste.

Serves 6 to 8.

Simple Lemon-Roasted Chicken
from *The Schwarzbein Principle Cookbook*

one 6-pound roasting chicken

2 crushed garlic cloves

juice of 1 lemon

1 sliced lemon

6 sprigs fresh rosemary

6 sprigs fresh parsley

sea salt, to taste

freshly ground black pepper, to taste

- Preheat oven to 450°.

- Rinse chicken under cold water, remove giblets, and pat dry with paper towels. Rub outside of chicken with 1 crushed garlic clove and lemon juice. Fill cavity with remaining garlic clove, lemon slices, rosemary, parsley, sea salt, and black pepper.

- Arrange chicken, breast side up, on a rack set in a roasting pan. Reduce heat to 400°. Bake about 1 hour and 15 minutes, or until tender and thigh juices run clear when pierced with a fork. Baste with pan juices.

- Allow chicken to rest at room temperature 10 to 15 minutes before carving.

Makes 6 servings.

Chicken with Sweet and Sour Sauce
from *Nourishing Traditions*

8 chicken breasts with skin on

1 cup fresh orange juice

1 cup fresh lemon juice

1 cup vinegar

2 tablespoons fresh ginger, peeled, and minced

2 tablespoons fresh garlic, peeled, and minced

½ teaspoon red chile pepper flakes

3 tablespoons olive oil

2 cups chicken stock

- Trim chicken breasts and pound lightly with the small-prong side of a meat hammer. Combine remaining ingredients, except olive oil and chicken stock, in a saucepan and bring to a boil. Reduce heat and simmer for several minutes. Allow to cool and stir in olive oil. Marinate the chicken breasts in this mixture for several hours or overnight. Remove from marinade and broil about 7 minutes per side. Keep warm in the oven while making sauce.

- Place marinade and stock in a saucepan and boil vigorously until sauce is reduced by half. To serve, slice the chicken breasts across the grain, arrange on individual plates, and spoon sauce over.

Makes 8 servings.

Baked Salmon
from *Nourishing Traditions*

1½ pounds salmon filet

½ lemon

2 tablespoons melted butter

1 tablespoon unbleached flour

¼ teaspoon paprika

½ teaspoon sea salt

· Lay salmon, skin side down, in a buttered Pyrex baking dish. Squeeze on lemon juice, then brush generously with butter. Sprinkle on flour and spread with your fingers to make a thin, even coat. Sprinkle on paprika and sea salt. Bake at 350° for 10 to 15 minutes or until salmon is almost, but not quite, cooked through. Place under broiler for just under 1 minute until flour coating becomes browned.

Makes 4 servings.

Mediterranean Shrimp
from *The Schwarzbein Principle Cookbook*

2 tablespoons olive oil

3 chopped garlic cloves

2 pounds raw shrimp, peeled and deveined

2 red or green bell peppers, cut into 1-inch squares

1 large eggplant (peeled, if desired) cut into 2-inch cubes

1 coarsely chopped medium red onion

⅓ cup olive oil

sea salt, to taste

freshly ground black pepper, to taste

2 medium tomatoes, cut into 1-inch cubes

1 tablespoon chopped fresh parsley

1 tablespoon fresh lemon juice

⅓ cup crumbled feta cheese

· Preheat oven to 425°.

· In a large nonstick skillet, heat oil over medium-high heat. When oil is hot, add garlic and shrimp and cook 2 to 5 minutes, or until shrimp are tender and turn pink. Remove from heat and set aside.

· In a large bowl, combine bell peppers, eggplant, onion, olive oil, and black pepper. Transfer to a greased baking sheet, spread in a single layer, and roast, stirring occasionally, until all vegetables are tender, about 20 minutes. Add tomatoes the last 5 minutes. Arrange all vegetables on a serving platter. Top with shrimp, parsley, lemon juice, and feta cheese. Taste, and adjust seasonings. Serve hot or at room temperature.

Makes 4 servings.

DRESSINGS, MARINADES, SAUCES, AND PESTOS

Basic Dressing
from *Nourishing Traditions*

1 teaspoon Dijon mustard, smooth or grainy

2 tablespoons plus 1 teaspoon raw wine vinegar

½ cup olive oil

1 tablespoon flax oil

• Dip a fork into the jar of mustard and transfer about 1 teaspoon to a small bowl. Add vinegar and mix around. Add olive oil in a thin stream, stirring all the while with the fork, until oil is well mixed or emulsified. Add flax oil and use immediately.

Makes about ¾ cup.

Dr. Hanley's Alkalinizing Buttermilk Dressing

1 cup buttermilk

3 tablespoon lemon juice

¼ teaspoon dry mustard

1½ teaspoon chopped fresh dill

This is an alkalinizing dressing to use on all types of salads.

• In a blender or food processor, blend all ingredients until smooth. Refrigerate 1 hour before serving. Season to taste.

Makes about 1½ cups.

California Coleslaw Dressing
from *The Schwarzbein Principle Cookbook*

½ cup mayonnaise

¼ cup red wine vinegar

½ teaspoon celery seed

Use on coleslaw or any mixed salad.

• In a blender or food processor, blend all ingredients until smooth; or place ingredients in a jar with tight-

1 teaspoon Dijon mustard

2 tablespoons minced fresh parsley

sea salt, to taste

freshly ground black pepper, to taste

fitting lid and shake vigorously until well blended. Taste, and adjust seasonings.

Makes about ¾ cup.

Creamy Vinaigrette
from *The Schwarzbein Principle Cookbook*

½ cup red wine vinegar

2 tablespoons Dijon mustard

2 tablespoons fresh lemon juice

1 minced garlic clove

1 cup olive oil

sea salt, to taste

freshly ground black pepper, to taste

Use on mixed greens, marinated vegetables, spinach, or potato salads.

· Combine all ingredients in a jar with a tight-fitting lid and shake vigorously until well blended. Taste, and adjust seasonings.

Makes about 1¾ cups.

Creamy Cucumber Marinade
from *The Schwarzbein Principle Cookbook*

⅔ cup whole sour cream

2 teaspoons minced fresh mint

2 teaspoons minced fresh parsley

2 teaspoons minced scallions

1 minced garlic clove

2 tablespoons fresh lemon juice

sea salt, to taste

freshly ground black pepper, to taste

Use on cucumber salad, or baked potatoes.

· In a medium bowl, using a fork, whisk dressing ingredients. Taste and adjust seasonings.

Makes about 1 cup.

Walnut Dressing
from *Nourishing Traditions*

2 tablespoons sherry vinegar

2 tablespoons unrefined walnut oil

6 tablespoons olive oil

Use on apple, pear, and green salads.

- Walnut oil is rich in Omega 3 fatty acids. Buy unrefined walnut oil in dark cans and store in the refrigerator. Place all ingredients in a bowl and stir with a fork.

Makes about ½ cup.

Cilantro Marinade
from *Nourishing Traditions*

1 bunch cilantro, chopped

juice of 1 lemon

3 garlic cloves, mashed

½ cup olive oil

¼ teaspoon black pepper

Delicious as a marinade for swordfish and eggplant.

- Mix all ingredients together.

Makes ½ cup.

Basil Pesto
from *The Schwarzbein Principle Cookbook*

2 cups packed fresh basil leaves

2 chopped garlic cloves

2 tablespoons raw pine nuts or raw walnuts

½ cup grated Parmesan cheese

⅓ cup olive oil

sea salt, to taste

freshly ground black pepper, to taste

dash cayenne pepper

Delicious with grilled fish, chicken, or baked potatoes.

- In a blender or food processor, puree all ingredients. Taste, and adjust seasonings.

Makes about ¾ cup.

Cilantro Pesto
from *The Schwarzbein Principle Cookbook*

2 bunches cilantro, coarsely chopped with stems removed

2 tablespoons fresh lime juice

½ cup roasted and chopped pumpkin seeds

½ cup grated Parmesan cheese

6 minced garlic cloves

½ cup olive oil

sea salt, to taste

freshly ground black pepper, to taste

Serve with grilled fish, chicken, or meat.

• In a blender or food processor, puree all ingredients. Taste and adjust seasonings. Store covered in refrigerator.

Makes about 1 cup.

Horseradish Sauce
from *The Schwarzbein Principle Cookbook*

2 tablespoons horseradish

¾ cup whole sour cream

1 tablespoon Dijon mustard

¼ teaspoon white vinegar

sea salt, to taste

freshly ground black pepper, to taste

Excellent with meat or poached fish.

• In a medium bowl, using a fork, combine all ingredients and mix well. Taste, and adjust seasonings. Refrigerate before serving.

Makes about 1 cup.

Coconut Curry Sauce
from *The Schwarzbein Principle Cookbook*

1 tablespoon unsalted butter

1½ tablespoons curry powder

2 minced garlic cloves

2 teaspoons peeled and finely minced fresh ginger

¼ teaspoon ground cardamom

1 teaspoon mustard seeds

Serve with grilled or baked fish, shrimp, chicken, or rice.

• In a medium saucepan, melt butter over medium-high heat. When butter is hot and bubbly, add curry powder, garlic, ginger, cardamom, and mustard seeds. Reduce heat to low and sauté 2 to 3 minutes, until mustard seeds begin to pop.

¾ cup heavy cream

½ cup coconut milk

1 tablespoon shredded unsweetened coconut

1 tablespoon minced fresh cilantro

2 teaspoons minced fresh mint

freshly ground black pepper, to taste

sea salt, to taste

· Add cream, coconut milk, coconut, cilantro, mint, and black pepper. Mix well with a wooden spoon. Simmer gently 5 minutes, stirring until thickened and well mixed. Taste, and adjust seasonings.

Makes about 1½ cups.

SNACKS

When you are eating out in a restaurant, order enough so you can take some food with you to go and eat it later on for your snack. When you prepare meals, make enough for the following day to have as another meal or as a snack. I always carry a snack with me if I think I am going to be away from a good food source. Here is a recipe for an alkalinizing snack you can take wherever you go. The fruits and nuts in this recipe have both fat-burning and alkalinizing qualities.

Dr. Hanley's Alkalinizing Trail Mix

¼ cup chopped dried figs

¼ cup almonds

¼ cup walnuts

¼ cup pumpkin seeds

¼ cup apricots, raisins or dates—avoid using banana chips, which are high in sugar

¼ cup chia seeds

· Mix together and carry with you for a convenient snack.

Makes 1½ cups.

Spicy Mixed Nuts

from *The Schwarzbein Principle Cookbook*

3 tablespoons olive oil

2 minced garlic cloves

½ teaspoon ground cumin

1 teaspoon curry powder

1 teaspoon low-sodium tamari soy sauce

dash red pepper flakes

½ teaspoon chili powder

1 cup whole raw almonds

1 cup whole raw cashews

1 cup raw pecan halves

1 cup whole raw peanuts

sea salt, to taste

· Preheat oven to 350º. In a large skillet, heat oil over medium heat. When oil is hot, add garlic and sauté until softened, about 10 seconds. Add cumin, curry powder, soy sauce, red pepper flakes, and chili powder. Stir well. Add mixed nuts and stir until thoroughly coated with spices.

· Transfer nut mix to a baking sheet. Bake 15 to 20 minutes, stirring frequently to bake evenly. Remove from oven and cool. Add salt to taste. Store in an airtight container.

Makes about 4 cups.

Chicken Liver Paté

from *Nourishing Traditions*

3 tablespoons butter

1 pound chicken or duck livers, or a combination

½ pound mushrooms, washed, dried, and coarsely chopped

1 bunch green onions, chopped

⅔ cup dry white wine or vermouth

1 clove garlic, mashed

½ teaspoon dry mustard

¼ teaspoon dried dill

¼ teaspoon dried rosemary

1 tablespoon lemon juice

½ stick butter, softened

sea salt

· Melt butter in a heavy skillet. Add livers, onions, and mushrooms and cook, stirring occasionally, for about 10 minutes until livers are browned. Add wine, garlic, mustard, lemon juice, and herbs. Bring to a boil and cook, uncovered, until the liquid is gone. Allow to cool. Process in a food processor with softened butter. Season to taste. Place in a crock or mold and chill well.

Makes 12 to 18 servings.

Nancy Deville's Favorite Deviled Eggs

6 hard-boiled eggs

4 tablespoons mayonnaise

2 teaspoons Dijon mustard

sea salt, to taste

freshly ground black pepper, to taste

paprika, for garnish

- To hard-boil eggs, place eggs in a saucepan and cover with cold water. Bring to a boil uncovered. Allow to boil for 1 minute, then cover, remove from heat and let sit undisturbed for 10 minutes. Rinse eggs under cold water.

- Peel eggs and cut in half lengthwise. Remove yolks. In a medium bowl, add mayonnaise, yolks, and mustard. Mash with fork until smooth. Season with salt and pepper to taste.

- Using a small teaspoon, fill egg white cavities with a dollop of egg mixture. Garnish with paprika.

Makes 12 halves.

Power Drinks

*Sixteen recipes
for power drinks*

Power drinks, especially made with green food, are wonderful sources of nutrients. But a power drink is not enough to keep you going all morning. Be sure to follow your power drink with a balanced breakfast within two hours—or have a power drink as prebreakfast starter or as a snack. Use protein powders that contain between 15 and 20 grams of protein per serving and preferably not more than 5 grams of carbohydrate. Servings are measured by the scoop that is enclosed in the container by the manufacturer.

Essential fatty acid blends are formulated to provide a healthy daily dose of Omega 3 and Omega 6 oils. The further you have progressed through the stages of burnout, the greater will be your need for EFAs. There are numerous healthy blends of EFAs at your health food store. You will either find them in capsules or bottled and refrigerated. If you are making power drinks, the easiest way to include good EFAs is to add 1 teaspoon or 1 tablespoon to your power drink. If you are not drinking power drinks, two to four capsules a day will provide you with your EFAs.

You can find super green food, stabilized rice bran, and protein powder at your health food store, or you can purchase a premixed formula. See page 355 for product references.

Blend the following recipes in a blender, add water or ice to taste. These recipes contain about 15 to 20 grams of carbohydrate.

Basic Protein Power Drink

8 ounces water

4 ounces raw milk or coconut milk

¼ piece of fruit

1 teaspoon to 1 tablespoon essential fatty acid blend

½ scoop protein powder

1 scoop super green food

1 scoop stabilized rice bran

¼ teaspoon extract of your choice—vanilla, almond, ginger, coffee

Strawberries 'n' Cream Protein Power Drink

6 to 8 ounces water

2 to 4 ounces coconut milk

7 frozen strawberries

1 teaspoon to 1 tablespoon essential fatty acid blend

1 scoop protein powder

1 scoop super green food

1 scoop stabilized rice bran powder

vanilla to taste

Almond Butter Power Drink

4 ounces plain whole cow or goat yogurt

6 ounces water and ½ cup crushed ice

1 teaspoon to 1 tablespoon essential fatty acid blend

1 tablespoon organic almond butter

½ scoop protein powder

1 scoop super green food

1 scoop stabilized rice bran powder

Cappuccino Power Drink

4 ounces plain cow or goat yogurt

6 ounces water and ½ cup crushed ice

1 teaspoon to 1 tablespoon essential fatty acid blend

½ scoop protein powder

1 scoop super green food

1 scoop stabilized rice bran powder

½ to 1 teaspoon coffee extract

Cinnamon Apple Protein Power Drink

8 ounces water

½ apple

1 teaspoon to 1 tablespoon essential fatty acid blend

1 scoop protein powder

1 scoop super green food

1 scoop stabilized rice bran powder

cinnamon to taste

Coconut Banana Protein Power Drink

6 to 8 ounces water

2 ounces coconut milk

⅓ frozen banana

1 teaspoon to 1 tablespoon essential fatty acid blend

1 scoop protein powder

1 scoop super green food

1 scoop stabilized rice bran powder

vanilla to taste

Wheat Germ Yogurt Power Drink

6 ounces water and ½ cup crushed ice

4 ounces plain whole cow or goat yogurt

1 teaspoon to 1 tablespoon essential fatty acid blend

2 tablespoons raw wheat germ

1 scoop protein powder

1 scoop super green food

1 scoop stabilized rice bran powder

almond extract to taste

Spicy Yogurt Power Drink

6 ounces water and ½ cup crushed ice

4 ounces plain cow or goat yogurt

1 teaspoon to 1 tablespoon essential fatty acid blend

1 scoop protein powder

1 scoop super green food

1 scoop stabilized rice bran powder

nutmeg and ginger to taste

Date Protein Power Drink

6 ounces water and ½ cup crushed ice

2 ounces coconut milk

2 dates

1 teaspoon to 1 tablespoon coconut oil

1 scoop protein powder

1 scoop super green food

1 scoop stabilized rice bran powder

Peach Protein Power Drink

6 ounces water and ½ cup crushed ice

½ diced fresh or frozen peach

1 teaspoon to tablespoon essential fatty acid blend

1 scoop protein powder

1 scoop super green food

1 scoop stabilized rice bran powder

Yogurt and Fig Power Drink

4 ounces plain cow or goat yogurt

4 ounces water and ½ cup crushed ice

1 teaspoon to 1 tablespoon essential fatty acid blend

1 fresh fig

½ scoop protein powder

1 scoop super green food

1 scoop stabilized rice bran powder

nutmeg and ginger to taste

Crunchy Power Drink

4 ounces plain cow or goat yogurt

4 ounces water and ½ cup crushed ice

¼ cup walnuts

1 tablespoon raw walnut oil

½ scoop protein powder

1 scoop super green food

1 scoop stabilized rice bran powder

Piña Colada Power Drink

6 ounces water and ½ cup crushed ice

4 ounces coconut milk

¼ cup cubed fresh pineapple

1 teaspoon to 1 tablespoon coconut oil

1 scoop protein powder

1 scoop super green food

1 scoop stabilized rice bran powder

Strawberry Yogurt Power Drink

4 ounces plain whole cow or goat yogurt

4 ounces water and ½ cup crushed ice

7 frozen strawberries

1 tablespoon essential fatty acid blend

½ scoop protein powder

1 scoop super green food

1 scoop stabilized rice bran powder

vanilla to taste

Dreamsicle Tofu Power Drink

4 ounces water and ½ cup crushed ice

4 ounces crumbled tofu

½ orange

1 teaspoon to 1 tablespoon essential fatty
acid blend

1 scoop protein powder

1 scoop super green food

1 scoop stabilized rice bran powder

⅛ teaspoon orange extract (optional)

Coconut Almond Power Drink

4 ounces water and ½ cup crushed ice

4 ounces coconut milk

10 almonds

1 tablespoon essential fatty acid blend

1 scoop protein powder

1 scoop super green food

1 scoop stabilized rice bran powder

almond extract to taste

Healthy Fats, Oils, and Essential Fatty Acids

A quick reference for good fats to eat and bad fats to avoid

Healthy saturated fats to eat at room temperature or to cook with

Butter	Cream	Palm kernel oil
Cheese	Eggs	Shea nut oil
Cocoa butter	Nutmeg oil	Sour cream
Cocoa butter or oil		

Healthy monounsaturated fats to eat at room temperature

Almond oil	Grape seed oil	Oat oil
Apricot kernel oil	Hazelnut oil	Rice bran oil
Avocado oil	Mustard oil	Sesame oil
Black currant oil		

Healthy monounsaturated fats to cook with

Chicken fat	Safflower oil if it is	cold-, pure-, or
Duck fat	cold-, pure-, or	expeller-pressed
Goose fat	expeller-pressed	Turkey fat
Olive oil	Sunflower oil if it is	

Cold-, pure-, or expeller-pressed polyunsaturated essential fatty acids to eat at room temperature

Almond oil	Borage oil	Salmon oil
Apricot oil	Herring oil	Sardine oil
Poppyseed oil	Menhaden (fish)	Walnut oil
Primrose oil	oil	Wheat germ oil
Flaxseed oil	Sesame seed oil	

Sources of Omega 3

Blue-green algae	Fish oil	Sardine oil
Chia seeds	Flaxseed oil	Spirulina (sea
Chlorella (sea	Hemp oil	algae)
algae)	Mackerel oil	Tuna fish
Dunalellia (sea	Pumpkin oil	Walnuts and oil
algae)	Salmon oil	

Sources of Omega 6

Butter	Fowl	Safflower oil
Cream	Grape seed oil	Sunflower oil
Eggs	Hemp oil	Turkey
Fish oil	Meat	Walnuts and oil
Flaxseed oil	Pumpkin oil	Wheat germ oil

Recommended Essential Fatty Acids

Essential fatty acid blends are formulated to provide a healthy
daily dose of Omega 3 and 6 oils. The further you have progressed through the stages of burnout, the greater will be your
need for EFAs. There are numerous healthy blends of EFAs at
your health food store. You will either find them in capsules or
bottled and refrigerated. If you are making power drinks, the easiest way to include good EFAs is to add 1 teaspoon or tablespoon
to your power drink. If you are not drinking power drinks, two to
four capsules a day will provide you with your EFAs.

> Essential Balance by Omega Oils
> Omega Twin by Barleans
> Udo's Choice
> Ultimate Oil by Nature's Secret
> Ultra Oil by Country Life
> Wild Alaskan Salmon Oil by Natural Factors

Never eat:

Heat-processed poly- and monounsaturated oils containing transfatty acids

Canola, unless it is cold-, pure-, or expeller-pressed

Mayonnaise made with heat-processed canola oil

Corn oil

Cottonseed oil

Peanut oil—healthy to eat on occasion if it is cold-, pure-, or expeller-pressed

Safflower oil, unless it is cold-, pure-, or expeller-pressed and mono-unsaturated

Sunflower oil, unless it is cold-, pure-, or expeller-pressed and monounsaturated

Soy oil

Avoid sources of hydrogenated, partially hydrogenated fats, and damaged polyunsaturated oils

Bottled salad dressings	Imitation mayonnaise	Non-dairy creamers
Chips	Imitation sour cream	Pressurized whipped cream
Cookies		
Corn oil	Margarine and other hydro-	Processed, junk, and fake foods
Cottonseed oil	genated fake	Sandwich spreads
Deep-fat fried foods	butter spreads	Shortening

Acid-Forming and Alkalinizing Foods

*What to eat more of and
what to avoid*

Acid-Forming Foods That Keep You in a State of Sympathetic Dominance

Processed food is made from real food that has been put through devitalizing chemical processes and is infused with chemicals and preservatives.

Beef jerky

Bologna

Cake, brownie, and cookie
  mixes

Canned foods containing
  chemicals

Canned or bottled tea and
  coffee drinks

Canned or jarred gravy and
  sauces containing
  chemicals

Canned soup containing
  chemicals

Hot dogs

Instant cereals and other
  instant foods

Jams, jellies, preserves, and marmalades with added sugar and chemicals

Low-fat yogurt with sugar or aspartame

Meats containing nitrates

Nuts and seeds roasted in hydrogenated oils

Pasta, bagels, pretzels, pizza, most breads, croissants, muffins, scones

Popcorn popped in hydrogenated oil

Potato chips

Tortilla chips processed in hydrogenated oils

TV dinners

White sugar

Junk foods contain very little real food—they are made of devitalized processed food, hydrogenated fats, chemicals, and preservatives.

Anything made with refined white flour

Candy

Canned breakfast drinks

Cereals (cold, sugary)

Doughnuts

Drive-through foods

Fried food

Low calorie foods

Low-fat foods

Pork skins

Powdered pudding mixes and pudding snacks

Sodas, especially those containing caffeine and sugar substitutes

Some ice cream products

Store-bought cookies

Sugary snack foods

Syrups—fudge, corn, high-fructose corn syrup

Toaster pastries

Fake foods are made primarily of chemicals and often contain gums and sugar fillers that will increase your risk of adrenal burnout.

Aspartame

Bacon bits

Barbecue sauces

Bottled salad dressing, especially diet dressings

Bouillon

Butter spreads (imitation)

Cheese (imitation)

Dehydrated soups

Egg substitutes
Flavor enhancers
Hoisin sauce
Hydrogenated
  oils
Instant coffee
Instant meals—
  liquid break-
  fasts, dried
  noodle soups
Ketchup
Margarine
Marshmallow
  cream
Mayonnaise
  (imitation)
Meat extender
Meat tenderizer
Microwaveable and
  other imitation
  food snacks
Non-dairy
  creamers
Oyster sauce
Packaged food
  helpers
Powdered fruit
  drinks
Powdered, canned,
  or bottled mixes
  for making alco-
  holic drinks
Relishes
Saccharin
Sandwich spreads
Shortening
Sour cream
  (imitation)
Whipped cream
  (artificial)
Worcestershire
  sauce

Miscellaneous acid-forming substances

Alcohol
Chemicals such as food addi-
  tives; household cleaners;
  garden poisons; flea and
  tick poisons; cigarettes,
  cigars, and other nicotine
  products; self-care products
  made with chemicals
Drugs, including over-the-
  counter and prescription
Aspartame
Caffeine
Cocoa and chocolate
Condiments such as ketchup
  and other products con-
  taining chemicals and
  sugar
Flavorings
Pesticides and other environ-
  mental toxins
Preservatives in foods
Saccharin
Tobacco
White sugar

Acid-forming fruit-based foods

Canned and/or sugared fruits
Dried, sulfured, glazed fruits
Preserves and jellies
Sorbet

Acid-forming grain-based foods

Refined flour products made from wheat, rye, barley, oat, or corn flour	Cornmeal	Pastry
	Corn flakes	Pies
	Crackers	Pizza
	Doughnuts	Starch
	Dumplings	White rice
Bread	Macaroni	
Cakes	Pasta	

Acid-forming dairy products

Ice cream	Homogenized and pasteurized milk	Sherbet
Custards		

Acid-forming nuts

Peanuts and other nuts roasted in hydrogenated fats

Alkaline-Forming Foods That Promote a Healthy Parasympathetic State
Alkaline-forming vegetables

Artichokes	Carrots	Dill
Asparagus	Celery	Eggplant
Barley grass	Cauliflower	Endive
Beans—green, lima, string, sprouts	Chard	Garlic
	Chlorella (sea algae)	Horseradish
Beets	Chicory	Jerusalem artichoke
Broccoli	Chives	Kale
Brussels sprouts	Collards	Leek
Cabbage—red and white	Cucumber	Legumes—except peanuts and
	Dandelion greens	

lentils, which are acidic
Lettuce
Mushrooms—maitake, shiitake, reishi
Okra
Olives
Onions
Parsley
Parsnips
Peas
Peppers
Potatoes
Pumpkin
Radish
Rhubarb
Rutabaga
Sauerkraut
Soy beans and sprouts
Spinach
Spirulina
Sprouts
Turnips
Water chestnut
Watercress
Wheat grass
Winter squash
Zucchini

Alkaline-forming fruits

Apples and cider
Apricots
Avocado
Bananas
Berries
Cantaloupe
Carob
Cherries
Citron
Cranberries
Currents
Dates
Figs—very high alkaline
Grapes
Grapefruit
Guavas
Kumquats
Lemons
Limes
Mangoes
Melons
Nectarines
Oranges
Papayas
Peaches
Pears
Persimmons
Pineapple
Plums
Pomegranates
Prunes
Quinces
Raisins
Strawberries
Tangerines
Tomatoes
Watermelon

Alkaline-forming dairy

Acidophilus
Buttermilk
Milk—raw, human, goat, cow
Whey
Yogurt

Alkaline-forming nuts

Sprouted seeds	Coconut	Sesame seeds
Almonds	Flaxseeds	Squash seeds
Chestnuts	Pumpkin seeds	Sunflower seeds

Alkaline-forming herbs and spices

All herbs such as	basil, balm,	Curry
marjoram,	bergamot,	Ginger
oregano, rose-	savory, tarragon,	Miso
mary, sage,	bay leaf, dill,	Mustard
mint, parsley,	fennel	Pepper
cilantro, chervil,	Baking soda	Sea salt
chives, thyme,	Cinnamon	

Alkaline-forming miscellaneous

Agar (sea algae)	Honey	Raw molasses
Alfalfa products	Kelp	Yeast cakes

Alkaline-forming beverage

Teas—alfalfa, clover, green, mint, sage, strawberry
Water

Alkaline-forming cereals

Millet	Buckwheat

Music for Calming the Central Nervous System

Music and positive imagery for relaxation and sleep

Don Campbell, founder of the Institute of Music, Health and Education and author of *The Mozart Effect* (Avon) and *The Mozart Effect for Children* (William Morrow), offered these guidelines for specific music to listen before going to bed.

Music for relaxation

- *Music for The Mozart Effect,* II (Spring Hill)

- *Gregorian Chant, Gregorian Sampler, Solesmes* (Paraclete Press)

- *Rosa Mystica* by Therese Schroeder-Sheker (Celestial Harmonies)

- *Sunsinger* by Paul Winter (Living Music)

- *Essence CD* by Don Campbell (Spring Hill)

- *Relax with the Classics,* III, *Pastorale* (Lind)

Music for deep rest and meditation

- *Thursday Afternoon* by Brian Eno (Sony)

- *Music for Airports* by Brian Eno (EMI)

- *Deep Listening* by Pauline Oliveros (New Albion)

- *Dolphin Dreams* by Jonathan Goldman (Spirit Music)

- *Angels* by Don Campbell (MHE)

- *Relax with the Classics,* I, *Largo* (Lind)

- *Essence* by Don Campbell, *Runes* (Spring Hill)

You may want to browse the music store and discover music for relaxation such as:

- Slower Baroque pieces

- Mozart's works

- Impressionist music—Debussy, Fauré, and Ravel

- Romantic music—Schubert, Schuman, Chopin, and Liszt

- New Age music

- Environmental music

My personal favorites for relaxation are:

- *Timeless Motion* by Daniel Kobialka

- *Om Namah Shivaya* by Robert Gass

- *Medicine Flutes* by Carlos Nakai

Relaxation and guided imagery tapes work well for a lot of people by taking them through a step-down process to relaxation.

Positive imagery tapes that can help you relax

- *Creative Visualization* by Shakti Gwain

- *Healing Journey, Easing into Sleep, Letting go of Stress,* and *Rainbow Butterfly* by Emmett Miller

- *The Art of EveryDay Ecstasy* by Depak Chopra, M.D., and Margo Anand

- *Secrets of Your Own Healing Power* by Depak Chopra, M.D., and Wayne Dwyer

- *Meditations for Enhancing your Immune System* by Bernie Siegel, M.D.

- *Breathing, the Master Key to Self-Healing* by Andrew Weil, M.D.,

- *Why People Don't Heal and How They Can* by Carolyn Myss

Afterword

A Word for You
from Dr. Hanley

⌒

In my practice, many people have come to me and talked about how wonderful it would be to be young again. Although weight and other factors of aging are often issues, most people's primary complaint is that they feel old and tired.

Over the past twenty-five years, I have learned that although we cannot turn back our chronological clock, we can look and feel younger, more energetic, and happier. I have witnessed thousands of chronically tired and ill people of all ages regain and reclaim their vitality, health, and passion for life. This is what I wish for you.

Taking the time to read this book may be the most important investment you have made in a very long time. You have given yourself the opportunity to reflect on where you may be on the path toward adrenal burnout—and what you can do about it. If any single message made an impression on you, I hope you have learned that small changes can make a huge difference in your future health and happiness. Small changes add up.

Since you have twenty, thirty, and even fifty more years to live, you may as well live those years as a healthy, vital, active person. It is never too late to begin making healthy changes and to enjoy the results of those changes. I cannot promise that you will look twenty again. But

I can promise that you will feel and look better than you ever imagined possible.

Why stay tired of being tired when you can feel energetic and passionate about life again? I wish you energy to burn for a lifetime and the good health you have always dreamed of.

References for Ordering Products

Multiple vitamin/mineral supplements, herbs, therapeutic nutrients, amino acids, glandulars, and hormones definitely have their place in modern society. Now that the nutritional industry is big business, as in any big business, not all products are created equal. It is important to know your source so that you know the products you buy are the highest quality. Sometimes when natural therapies have failed it is because the product was poor in quality. Not every company is scrupulous about putting the nutrients listed on the label in each bottle. Just because a bottle may say 1,000 milligrams of vitamin C does not mean that it truly contains that amount of vitamin C.

Throughout this book I have listed formulas that I consider optimal. You can purchase these exact supplement formulas that have been specifically formulated for the five stages of burnout as well as a premixed super green drink all created by Metagenics at *adrenalburnout. com* or by calling 1-877-547-5499. I also recommend and trust products made by Ethical Nutrients, Solray, Rainbow Light, and New Chapter—which are all available in your health food store.

For more information or to purchase white noise machines:

Marpac
P.O. Box 3098
Wilmington, NC 28406

(800) 999-6962
Fax (910) 763-4219
www.marpac.com

For magnetic therapy treatment guidance for all health issues, practitioner education, and seminars and to order magnetic products:

Magnetizer Biomagnetic
  Research Institute
Cathy Moore, Director
P.O. Box 2130

Ventura, CA 93002
(805) 643-0007
website: *magnetizer.org*
email: *biomags@magnetizer.com*

For more information on Dr. Philpott's magnetic therapy research program:

William H. Philpott, M.D.
17171 S.E. 29th Street
Choctaw, OK 73020

(405) 390-3009
Fax (405) 390-3309

Mail order catalogs to order safe household and self-care products:

Allergy Relief Shop
(865) 522-2795 or
(800) 626-2810
www.allergyreliefshop.com

Alorex
(800) 447-1100
www.alorex.com

The Living Source
(254) 776-4878, (800) 662-8787
www.livingsource.com

Nigra Enterprises
(818) 889-6877
www.nigra.org

Real Goods
(800) 762-7325
www.realgoods.com

Appendix

B

Health
Practitioner
Referrals

**Organizations you can contact for physician
referrals in your area:**

American College for the
   Advancement in Medicine
P.O. Box 3427
(800) 532-3688 or
   (964) 583-7666
www.acam.org

American Association of
   Naturopathic Physicians
8201 Greensboro Drive, Suite
   300

McLeon, VA 22102
(703) 610-9037
www.naturopathic.org/welcome.html

American Preventive Medicine
   Association
P.O. Box 458
Great Falls, VA 22066
(703) 759-0662
www.apma.net

The Broda O. Barnes, M.D., Research Foundation, Inc. is a not-for-profit organization dedicated to education, research, and training in the field of metabolic balance and thyroid. Thyroid problems often have roots in adrenal burnout.

P.O. Box 110098
Trumbull, CT 06611
203-261-2101
(Fax) 203-261-3017
info@BrodaBarnes.org

Information on Adrenal Blood, Urine, and Saliva Testing

The adrenal reserve test in chapter 3 helped you assess your behaviors and symptoms that relate to adrenal burnout. Medical tests of your adrenal function can also be helpful in determining the condition of your adrenal glands. Adrenal tests come in the form of blood, urine, and saliva tests. All of these test only cortisol levels. Adrenaline is the body's response to emergency stress, while cortisol is the hormone that is released to handle long-term stress. At midnight your cortisol levels are the lowest. During the night, cortisol levels steadily rise to reach a peak level around the time that you are rising and starting to meet the challenges of your day. Cortisol levels peak at 8 A.M. and decline to their lowest level around 4 P.M., which is the time when daily stresses are supposed to subside. Those who have weakened adrenals will feel a dramatic slump or will unconsciously reach for sugar or caffeine between 3 and 5 P.M. when this decline occurs.

These tests can give you a glimpse into the health of your adrenal glands.

Blood Test

There are two blood tests that measure cortisol. One test measures cortisol output at the peak and low points, and the other gauges your adrenal reserve or your ability to produce cortisol.

The first cortisol blood test measures cortisol levels at 8 to 9 A.M., which is typically the high point of adrenal output, and/or at 4 P.M., which is the typical low point of adrenal output.

Adrenal reserve is the capacity of your adrenal glands to respond to physical or emotional pressure by releasing cortisol from the adrenal cortex. If your adrenal reserve is healthy, your adrenal cortex will be able to repeatedly secrete cortisol in amounts that meet your body's demand. If your adrenal reserve is low, your adrenal cortex will not be able to sustain the secretion of cortisol necessary to provide the systems of your body with adequate direction. A lack of adrenal cortex reserve will manifest as fatigue, depression, irritability, cravings, and immune dysfunction, to name a few key signs and symptoms.

The blood test to measure adrenal reserve involves drawing blood at eight to ten A.M. to get a baseline cortisol level. Then you will be given a shot of cortrisyn, which is an adrenal releasing factor-like substance that stimulates your adrenals. One-half hour later your blood will be drawn again to see how much more cortisol your adrenals are capable of releasing under this standard stimulus. Your second cortisol level has to more than double the original baseline level to be considered an adequate amount of adrenal reserve, regardless of the initial baseline.

Urine Test

The twenty-four-hour urine test measures your total adrenal output of cortisol. This test requires that you collect and refrigerate *all* your urine during a twenty-four-hour period. This test must be done through your physician.

The twenty-four-hour urine test is more comprehensive than the first blood test, which only measures cortisol output at its peak and low point.

Saliva test

Saliva testing measures the rise-and-fall pattern of your cortisol output. Many saliva testing companies will have you collect saliva specimens every four hours; others will ask you to collect specimens every six hours. Both approaches are valid but give you slightly different windows to look at the same information. This test is the only test you do not need a medical doctor for. It is well researched. In fact, for adrenal burnout, this is my preferred test.

Because health insurance will only pay for tests your doctor orders, ask your doctor to order the saliva test.

Dr. Michael Borkin, director of the Sabre Science saliva testing laboratory, had this to say about saliva testing. "I have found the most effective way to determine the level of person's accumulated stress is to analyze their body's response to stress throughout a twenty-four-hour period of time. This can be accomplished by testing saliva every four hours throughout a twenty-four-hour period. The advantages to using saliva instead of blood are many. Saliva testing can be done without altering one's schedule and within one's normal everyday environment. Being in one's customary environment allows for the optimal representation of how the individual's body responds to stress. Unlike blood, which is the equivalent of a snapshot in time, saliva testing allows for a three-dimensional representation, like a video of twenty-four hours. Using a saliva test to establish a baseline (starting point) will give you a reference point so that you can begin to take steps to break out of your destructive patterns."

If your doctor will not order the test for you, she or he may be willing to order the cortrisyn stimulation test described earlier, which is my second choice.

Be aware that any of your test results might say that your adrenal reserve is healthy, when it really is not. Traditional medical interpretations are based on a set range of readings that are deemed normal as opposed to what may be normal for *you*. It is always advisable to factor your symptoms along with medical tests to come up with a sound diagnosis of your condition. Do not disregard your symptoms even if medical tests tell you that you are healthy.

Most doctors do not recognize adrenal burnout until it becomes Addison's disease—a rare condition in which the adrenal glands fail to secrete stress hormones caused by infectious disease or from trauma such as a car accident, gunshot, or knife wound.

Traditional Western medicine is oriented toward treating disease. Nontraditional Western medicine practitioners, such as naturopaths, herbalists, nutritionists, acupuncturists, and chiropractors, recognize the shades of gray between health and disease and help you create a path to greater health before disease is inevitable. If your physician is not already comfortable with the idea of adrenal burnout, it may be in your best interest to find a health practitioner who is familiar with this condition. A true health care partner will be interested in using a number of tests and treatments to support your efforts to be healthy.

The labs I recommend for saliva testing are:

Great Smokies Diagnostic
  Laboratory
63 Zillicoa St.
Asheville, NC 28801
800 522-4762
http://www.gsdl.com

David Zava
ZRT Laboratory
12505 NW Cornell Road
Portland, OR 97213
(503) 469-0741

For more information on hair analysis:

Great Smokies Diagnostic
  Laboratory
63 Zillicoa St.
Asheville, NC 28801
800 522-4762
http://www.gsdl.com

References for Further Reading

Chapter 4

The Schwarzbein Principle by Diana Schwarzbein, M.D., and Nancy Deville (Health Communications) is a comprehensive book on achieving a healthy metabolism and weight loss by eating balanced meals of real, whole foods. This book contains extensive carbohydrate guides for real foods. Available in bookstores or at amazon.com.

Most of the recipes in this book were taken from the following three cookbooks: *The Schwarzbein Principle Cookbook* and *The Schwarzbein Principle Vegetarian Cookbook* by Diana Schwarzbein, M.D., Nancy Deville, and Evelyn Jacob Jaffe (Health Communications) focus on appetizing, easy-to-prepare, balanced meat-based and vegetarian meals using real, whole foods. Evelyn Jacob Jaffe, who developed the recipes, is an authority on low-carbohydrate cuisine. Available in bookstores and at amazon.com.

Nourishing Traditions: The Cookbook that Challenges Politically Correct Nutrition and the Diet Dictocrats by Sally Fallon and Mary G. Enig, Ph.D. (New Trends): Nutrition researcher Sally Fallon united the wisdom of the ancients with the latest independent and accurate scientific research to create balanced recipes using real, whole foods that your grandmother would have made pre–World War II. Available at *www.newtrendspublishing.com,* or (877) 707-1776.

Know Your Fats: The Complete Primer for Understanding the Nutrition of Fats, Oil and Cholesterol and *Transfatty Acids in the Food Supply* by Dr. Mary Enig (Bethesda Press) *www.bethesdapress.com*. Dr. Enig's website, *www.knowyourfats.com* provides the latest information about fats and oils.

"The Oiling of America" by Dr. Enig and Sally Fallon—download from *westonaprice.org*—is an easy-to-read comprehensive report on the history of the lipid hypothesis and the many scientific studies that have since disproven this theory.

Attention Deficit Disorder by Dr. Jesse Hanley (Impact) is a complete guide on how to treat ADD and ADHD naturally. Available at amazon.com.

Chapter 6

Power Sleep: The Revolutionary Program That Prepares Your Mind for Peak Performance by James Maas, M.D. (Villard), provides further reading for those interested in learning more about the power of sleep.

Yoga: The Spirit and Practice of Moving into Stillness by Erich Schiffmann (Pocket Books) and his award-winning video "Yoga Mind and Body," with Ali Mac-Graw—which is great for beginners through intermediate—are available in video stores, bookstores, and at amazon.com.

How to Stop Worrying and Start Living by Dale Carnegie (Pocket Books) is extremely helpful for those who are prone to needless worry. Available in bookstores or at amazon.com.

The Mozart Effect (Avon), and *The Mozart Effect for Children* (William Morrow) by Don Campbell are guides to the pleasures and health benefits of music. Available in bookstores or amazon.com.

Chapter 10

The Relaxation Response by Herbert Benson, M.D. (Avon), is a book that pioneered meditation in this country. Available on amazon. Com.

Magnetic Therapy by William H. Philpott, M.D. (Future Medicine Publishers), is an explanation of the use of magnetic therapy and discusses Dr. Philpott's research on magnetic therapy. Available in bookstores and at www.alternative.com.

Chapter 11

Diet for a Poisoned Planet by David W. Steinman (Freedom Press) is a well-researched, thoroughly documented book on the perils of environmental toxins. Available in bookstores and at amazon.com.

The Safe Shopper's Bible: A Consumer's Guide to Nontoxic Household Products, Cosmetics, and Food by David W. Steinman, M.A., and Samuel S. Epstein, M.D. (Macmillan). This book contains extensive lists of brand-named products that are safe and of those that are toxic and carcinogenic. Available in bookstores and at amazon.com.

Living Healthy in a Toxic World: Simple Steps to Protect You and Your Family from Everyday Chemicals, Poisons and Pollution by David W. Steinman and R. Michael Wisner (Berkeley), explains how you can further protect yourself from toxins. Available in bookstores and at amazon.com.

Cross Currents (Tarcher) and *The Body Electric* by Robert Becker, M.D. (Quill). Geared toward the scientifically minded; an electropollution authority explains how electricity impacts our world. Available in bookstores and at amazon.com.

Whole Body Dentistry: Discover the Missing Piece to Better Health by Mark A. Breiner, D.D.S., and *Fluoride the Aging Factor: How to Recognize and Avoid the Devastating Effects of Fluoride* by John Yiamouyiannis (Health Action Press) provide more information on the dangers of silver fillings and fluoride. Available at amazon.com.

Notes

Chapter 2

Stout, Robert W., "Insulin and Atheroma 20-year Perspective." *Diabetes Care* 13, no. 6 (June 1990): 631.

Chapter 4

Geoffrey Cowley, "Generation XXL," *Newsweek* (3 June 2000): 40–47.

M. Enig, "Trans Fatty Acids in the Food Supply: A Comprehensive Report Covering 60 Years of Research," Enig Associates, Inc.: Maryland ed. (1995):4–8; D. Groom, "Population Studies of Atherosclerosis," *Annals of Internal Medicine* 55, no. 1 (July 1995): 51–62; W. F. Enos, F. R. Senti, et al., "Health Aspects of Dietary Trans Fatty Acids," Life Sciences Research Office (LSRO) of Federation of American Societies for Experimental Biology (FASEB), Bethesda Maryland: 1985; W. F. Enos, and O. J. Pollak, "Diet and Atherosclerosis," *Lancet* 1, no. 444 (1959); R. E. Olson, "Evolution of Ideas about the Nutritional Value of Dietary Fat: Introduction," *Journal of Nutrition* 128 (1998): 421S–425S.

L. D. Lawson, and F. Kummerow. "B-Oxidation of the Coenzyme A Esters of Vaccenic, Elaidic and Petroselaidic Acids by Rat Heart Mitochondria," *Lipids* 14 (1979): 501–503.

P. J. Jones et al., "Interaction of Dietary Fat Saturation and Cholesterol Level on Cholesterol Synthesis Measured Using Deuterium Incorporation," *Journal of Lipid Research* 35 (1994): 1093–1101.

Harvard Health Letter, "Eggcellent News" 24, no.9 (July 1999): 8; *Harvard Heart Letter,* "Good News for Egg Lovers" 12 (9 August 1999): 4.

M. G. Enig, et al., "Dietary Fat and Cancer Trends—A Critique," Federation Proceedings for Federation of American Societies for Experimental Biology (FASEB) 37, no. 9 (July 1978): 2215–2220; T. H. Applewhite, "Statistical 'Correlations' Relating Trans Fats to Cancer: A Commentary," Federation Proceedings for FASEB 38, no. 11 (October 1979): 2435–2439; S. M. Grundy, "Cholesterol and Coronary Heart Disease: A New Era," *JAMA* 256, no. 20 (28 November 1986): 2849–2858; W. C. Willett, et al., "Intake of Trans Fatty Acids and Risk of Coronary Heart Disease among Women," *Lancet* 341 (1993): 581–585; a general review of citations for problems with polyunsaturate consumption is found in E. R. Pinckney and C. Pinckney, *The Cholesterol Controversy*, Sherbourne Press: Los Angeles (1973), 127–131; Mary G. Enig, *Trans Fatty Acids in the Food Supply: A Comprehensive Report Covering Sixty Years of Research*, 2nd ed., Enig Associates: Maryland, 1995.

Mary G. Enig, "Lauric Oils as Antimicrobial Agents: Theory of Effect, Scientific Rationale, and Dietary Applications as Adjunct Nutritional Support for HIV-infected Individuals in Nutrients and Foods in AIDS," in R. R. Watson, ed., CRC Press: Boca Raton, FL (1998) 81–97.

A general review of citations for problems with polyunsaturate consumption is found in E. R. Pinckney and C. Pinckney, *The Cholesterol Controversy*, Sherbourne Press: Los Angeles (1973), 127–131.

C. V. Felton, et al., "Dietary Polyunsaturated Fatty Acids and Composition of Human Aortic Plaques," *Lancet* 344 (1994): 1195.

A detailed explanation of how polyunsaturates cause cancer is found in the *American Journal of Medicine* 35 (August 1963): 143; and *Medical Tribune* (29 September 1971); the relationship of polyunsaturates to breast cancer is discussed in *Canadian Medical Association Journal* 98 (23 March 1968): 590.

Michael Schmidt, *Smart Fats*. Frog: Berkeley, CA (1997).

Liver damage from polyunsaturates has been shown by Dr. Nicolas R. DiLuzio (of Tulane University in New Orleans), *Modern Medicine* (14 June 1971); Dr. W.O. Caster, *Life Sciences* 9 (1971): 81; and Dr. S. A. Norkin, *Archives of Pathology* 83 (January 1967): 31. Evidence of liver damage directly from the use of corn oil is in the *Archives of Pathology* 82 (December 1966): 596; details of the toxicity of corn oil, including death, are in *Journal of Clinical Pharmacology* (May/June 1969): 137.

A. A. Nanji, et al., *Gastroenterology* 109, no. 2 (August 1995): 547–54; Y. S. Cha, D. S. Sachan, *Journal of the American College of Nutrition* 13, no. 4 (August 1994): 338–343.

Michael Schmidt, *Smart Fats*. Frog: Berkeley, California, 1997.

M. W. Louwman, M. van Duddelsdorp, F. J. van de Vijver, et al., "Signs of Impaired Cognitive Function in Adolescents with Marginal Cobalamin Status," *American Journal of Clinical Nutrition* 72, no. 3 (2000 September): 762–769.

Solomon, H. Katz, "Food and Biocultural Evolution: A Model for the Investigation of Modern Nutritional Problems," *Nutritional Anthropology,* Alan R. Liss Inc. (1987) 50; S. J. Van-Rensburg, et al., "Nutritional Status of African Populations Predisposed to Esophageal Cancer," *Nutr-Cancer* 4 (1983): 206–216; P. B. Moser, et al., "Copper, Iron, Zinc and Selenium Dietary Intake and Status of Nepalese Lactating Women and Their Breast-fed Infants," *American Journal of Clinical Nutrition* 47 (April 1988): 729–734; B. F. Harland, et al., "Nutritional Status and Phytate: Zinc and Phytate X Calcium: Zinc Dietary Molar Ratios of Lacto-ovo-vegetarian Trappist Monks: 10 Years Later," *Journal of American Diet Association* 88 (December 1988): 1562–1566.

Chapter 5

Christopher P. Neck and Kenneth H. Cooper, "The Fit Executive: Exercise and Diet Guidelines for Enhancing Performance." *Academy of Management Executive* 14, no. 2 special issue, "Executive Health" (May 2000): 72–83.

E. E. Calle, E. Eugenia, M. J. Thun, et al., "Body-mass Index and Mortality in a Prospective Cohort of U.S. Adults," *New England Journal of Medicine* 341 (1999)1097–1105; S. N. Blair, H. W. Kohl, R. S. Paffenbarger, Jr., et al., "Physical Fitness and All-cause Mortality: A Prospective Study on Healthy Men and Women," *Journal of American Medical Association* 262, no.17 (1989): 2395-2401; S. N. Blair, H. W. Kohl, C. E. Barlow, et al., "Changes in Physical Fitness and All-cause Mortality: A Prospective Study on Healthy and Unhealthy Men," *JAMA* 273, no. 14 (1995): 1093–1098.

R. J. Shepard, "Do Work-site Exercise and Health Programs Work?" *Physician and Sports Medicine* 27 (1999):48–72; D. R. Frew and N. S. Brunning, "Improved Productivity and Job Satisfaction through Employees Exercise Programs," *Hospital Material Management Quarterly* 9 (1988): 62–69; L. R. Gettman, "The Effect of Employee Physical Fitness on Job Performance," *Personnel Administrator* (November 1980): 41–61.

N. S. Lupinacci, R. E. Rikli, C. J. Jones, et al., "Age and Physical Activity Effects Reaction Time and Digit Symbol Substitution Performance in Cognitive Active Adults," *Research Quarterly for Exercise and Sport* 64, no. 2 (1993): 144–151.

D. Ornish, S. E. Brown, L. W. Scherwitz, et al., "Can Lifestyle Changes Reverse Coronary Heart Disease?" *Lancet* 336, no. 21 (July 1990): 129–133.

M. B. Higginbotham, K.G. Morris, R. S. Williams, et al., "Physiologic Basis for the Age Related Decline in Aerobic Work Capacity," *American Journal of Cardiology* 57 (1986): 1374–1379; P. Haber, M. K. Honiger, and M. Neiderberger, "Effects on Elderly People 67–76 Years of Age of Three Month Endurance Training on a Bicycle Ergometer," *European Heart Journal* 5 (1984): supplement E, 37–39. J. Strovas, "Chronic Illness Need Not Deter Elderly Exercisers," *Physician and Sports Medicine* 18, no. 2 (1990): 20.

M. Sinaki, "Exercise and Osteoporosis," *Archives of Physical Medicine and Rehabilitation* 70 (March 1989): 220–229; J. A. Work, "Strength Training: A Bridge to Independence for the Elderly," *Physician and Sports Medicine* 17, no. 11 (1989): 134–138.

Chapter 7

James Maas, *Power Sleep: The Revolutionary Program That Prepares Your Mind for Peak Performance,* New York: Villard (1998).

P. Monteleone, M. Maj, L. Beinat, et al., "Blunting by Chronic Phosphatidylserine Administration of the Stress-induced Activation of the Hypothalamo-pituitary-adrenal Axis in Healthy Men," *European Journal of Clinical Pharmacology* 42, no. 4 (1992): 385–388; P. Monteleone, L. Beinat, C. Tanzillo, et al., "Effects of Phosphatidylserine on the Neuroendocrine Response to Physical Stress in Humans,"*Neuroendocrinology* 52, no. 3 (September 1990): 243–248; Eve Van Cauter, Karine Spiegel, Rachel Leproult, "Impact of Sleep Debt on Metabolic and Endocrine Function," *Lancet* 354 (23 October 1999): 1435–1439.

David Steinman, *Diet for a Poisoned Planet,* New York: Harmony Books (1990).

French physician Alfred Tomatis, M.D., devoted his life to researching what he called the "Mozart Effect." The Mozart Effect is defined by Don Campbell as "an inclusive term signifying the transformational powers of music in health, education and wellbeing." Don Campbell, *The Mozart Effect,* New York: Avon Books (1997), p. 14.

A. M. Kumar, F. Tims, D. G. Cruess, et al., "Music Therapy Increases Serum Melatonin Levels in Patients with Alzheimer's Disease," *Alternative Therapies in Health and Medicine* 5, no. 6 (November 1999): 49–57.

Claire V. Wilson and Leona S. Aiken, "The Effect of Intensity Levels upon Physiological and Subjective Affective Response to Rock Music," *Journal of Music Therapy* 14 (1977): 60–77.

J. F. Byers and K. A. Smyth, "Effect of a Music Intervention on Noise Annoyance, Heart Rate, and Blood Pressure in Cardiac Surgery Patients," *American Journal of Critical Care* 6, no. 3 (May 1997): 183–91.

L. Salk, " The Importance of the Heartbeat Rhythm to Human Nature: Theo-rectical, Clinical and Experimental Observations," *Proceedings of the Third World Congress of Psychiatry* (1961); L. Salk, "Mother's Heartbeat as an Im-printing Stimulus," *Transactions of the New York Academy of Sciences* 24 (1962): 753–763.

Chapter 8

R. J. Wurtman and J. J. Wurtman, "Brain Serotonin, Carbohydrate-craving, Obe-sity and Depression," *Obesity Research* (November 3): supplement 4, 477S–480S.

Ali A. Mokdad, "Diabetes Trend in the U.S.: 1990–1998," *Diabetes Care* 23, no. 9 (September 2000).

J. P. Després, et al., "Hyperinsulinemia as an Independent Risk Factor for Is-chemic Heart Disease," *New England Journal of Medicine* 334, no. 15 (11 April 1996): 952.

J. E. Spiegel, et al., "Safety and Benefits of Fructooligosaccharides as Food Ingre-dients," *Food Technology* (1994): 85–89; K. Yamashita et al., "Effects of Fruc-tooligosaccharides on Blood Glucose and Serum Lipids in Diabetic Subjects," *Nutrition Research* 4 (1984): 961–966.

Chapter 11

David Steinman, *Diet for a Poisoned Planet,* New York: Harmony Books (1990).

H. H. Schaumburg, R. Byck, R. Gerstl, and J. H. Mashman, "Monosodium L-glutamate: Its Pharmacology and Role in the Chinese Restaurant Syndrome," *Science* 163(1969): 826–828; R. A. Kenney and C. S. Tidball, "Human Suscepti-bility to Oral Monosodium L-glutamate," *Amercian Journal of Clinical Nutrition* 25 (1972): 140–146.

S. W. Ewen and A. Pusztai, "Health Risks of Genetically Modified Foods," *Lancet* 354 (21 August 1999): 684.

S. W. Ewen and A. Pusztai, "Effect of Diets Containing Genetically Modified Pota-toes Expressing Galanthus Nivalis Lectin on Rat Small Intestine," *Lancet* 354 (16 October 1999): 1353–1354.

A. Blair, "Cancer Risks Associated with Agriculture: Epidemiologic Evidence," *Basic Life Science* 21 (1982): 93-111; G. K. Raabe and O. Wong, "Leukemia Mor-tality by Cell Type in Petroleum Workers with Potential Exposure to Ben-zene," *Environmental Health Perspective* 104 (December1996): supplement 6, 1381–1392; S. S. Epstein, "The Politics of Cancer: The Costs of Failure to Reg-ulate." Proceedings of the Warner-Lambert Science and Public Policy Colloquium, The University of Michigan, Collegiate Institute for Values and Science, 1–2 November 1980.

A. B. Graves, et al., "The Association between Aluminum-containing Products and Alzheimer's Disease," *Journal of Clinical Epidemilogy* 43, no. 1 (1990): 35–44.

National Center for Health Statistics, Center for Disease Control and Prevention, *Healthy People: Statistical Notes,* National Committee on Vital and Health Statistics, Office of Disease Prevention, Washington, D.C. (2000).

"Fluoridated Toothpaste to Carry Warning on Its Packaging," *Sun,* 9 January 1998. Based on the National Center for Disease Control issue that excessive use of fluoridated toothpaste is hazardous to your health and could result in poisoning; Mullenix et al.,"Neurotoxicity of Sodium Fluoride in Rats," *Neurotoxicology and Teratology* (1995); J. Colquhuom, "Why I Changed My Mind about Fluoridation," *Perspectives in Biology and Medicine* (1997): 411–416.

Robert O. Becker, *Cross Currents,* New York: Putnam (1990), pp. 243–247.

U.S. Department of Health and Human Services, Public Health Service National Toxicology Program, Environmental Health Information Service, National Institute of Environmental Health Sciences (NIEHS), National Institutes of Health, *Report on Carcinogens,* North Carolina (1998).

Katie Norris, *Magnetic Miracles,* California: Energy Essentials, (1999), p. 24.

F. L. Lorscheider, M. J. Vimy, and A. O. Summers, "Mercury Exposure from Silver Tooth Fillings: Emerging Evidence Questions a Traditional Dental Paradigm," *Journal of the Federation of American Societies for Experimental Biology* 9, no. 7 (April 1995): 504–508.

Stanley R. Saxe, D.M.D., "Dental Amalgam and Cognitive Functions in Older Women: Findings from the Nun Study," *Journal of the American Dental Association* 126 (November 1995): 1495–1501.

A. Chattopadhyay, T. Roberts, and R. Jervis, "Scalp Hair as a Monitor of Community Exposure to Lead," *Archives of Environmental Health* 32, no. 5 (1977): 226–236; T. Suzuki and R. Yamamoto, "Organic Mercury Levels in Human Hair with and without Storage for Eleven Years," *Bulletin of Environmental Contamination Toxicology* 28 (1982): 186–188; D. Airey, "Mercury in Human Hair Due to Environment and Diet: A Review," *Environmental Health Perspectives* 52 (1983): 303–316.

Chapter 12

L. S. Berk and S.A. Tan, et al., "Immune System Changes During Humor Associated with Laughter," *Clinical Research* 39 (1991): 124A; J. V. Basmajian, "The Elixir of Laughter," *Archives of Physical Medicine and Rehabilitation* 80, no. 5

(May 1999): 608; L. S. Berk, "Neuroendocrine and Stress Hormone Changes during Mirthful Laughter," *American Journal of Medicine* 298 (1989): 390–396; N. Cousins, *Anatomy of an Illness,* New York: Bantam (1991); Allen Klein, *Tribulations and All That: The Healing Power of Humor: Techniques for Getting Through Loss, Setbacks, Upsets, Disappointments, Difficulties, Trials, Tribulations, and All That,* New York: Putnam (1989), pp. 390–396.

General References

D. Kritchevsky, "Diet and Cholesteremia," *Lipids* 12 (1977): 49–52.

G. L. Blackburn, G. Kater and E. A. Mascioli, et al., "A Reevaluation of Coconut Oil's Effect on Serum Cholesterol and Atherogenesis," *Journal of Philippine Medical Association* 65 (1989): 144–152.

M. F. Dallman, A. M. Strack, and S. F. Arkana, et al., "Feast and Famine: Critical Role of Glucocorticoids with Insulin in Daily Energy Flow," *Front Neuroendocrinology* 14, no. 4 (1993): 303–347.

J. Raber, "Detrimental Effects of Chronic Hypothalamic-Pituitary-Adrenal Axis Activation from Obesity to Memory Deficits," *Molecular Neurobiology* 18, no.1 (1998): 1–22.

S. Luo, J. Luo, and A. H. Cincotta, "Chronic Ventomedial Hypothalamic Infusion of Norepinephrine and Serotonin Promotes Insulin Resistance and Glucose Intolerance," *Neuroendocrinology* 70 (1999): 460–465.

P. Bjorntorp, "Neuroendocrine Perturbations as a Cause of Insulin Resistance," *Diabetes Metabolic Research Review* 15, no. 6 (1999): 427–441.

D. Foster, "Insulin Resistance—A Secret Killer," *New England Journal of Medicine* 320 (1989): 733–734.

W. Jeffries, *Safe Uses of Cortisone,* Springfield, IL: Charles C. Thomas (1981).

M. A. Demitrack, "Chronic Fatigue Syndrome: A Disease of the Hypothalamic-Pituitary-Adrenal Axis. *Annals of Internal Medicine* 26, no.1 (1994): 1–5.

W. M. Jeffies, "Mild Adrenocortical Deficiency, Chronic Allergies, Autoimmune Disorders and the Chronic Fatigue Syndrome: A Continuation of the Cortisone Story," *Medical Hypothesis* 42, no. 3 (1994): 183–189.

C. Hiemke, R. Brunner, E. Hammes, et al., "Circadian Variations in Antigen-specific Proliferation of Human T lymphocytes and Correlation to Cortisol Production," *Pychoneuroendocrinology* 20 (1995): 335–342.

N. S. Goulding and P. M. Guyre, "Glucocorticoids, Lipocortins and the Immune Response," *Current Opinions in Immunology* 5 (1993): 108–113.

A. Guyton and J. Hall, *Textbook of Medical Physiology,* Philadephia: Saunders (1996), pp. 769–781.

M. H. Joseph and G. A. Kennett, "Stress-Induced Release of 5-HT in the Hippocampus and its Dependence on Increased Tryptophan Availability: An In Vivo Electrochemical Study," *Brain Research* 270 (1983): 281–287.

S. C. Stanford, *Monoamines in Response and Adaptation to Stress,* London: Academic Press (1993), pp. 24–30.

S. C. Stanford and P. Salmon, eds., *Stress from Synapse to Syndrome,* London: Academic Press (1993), pp. 24–30.

M. Maes and H. Meltzer, "The Serotonin Hypothesis of Major Depression," F. E. Bloom and D. J. Kupfer, eds., *Psychopharmacology: The Fourth Generation of Progress.* New York: Raven Press (1995): 933–944.

H. Anisman and R. M. Zacharko, "Depression as a Consequence of Inadequate Neurochemical Adaptation in Response to Stressors," *British Journal of Psychiatry* 160 (1992): 36–43.

F. G. Graeff, F. S. Guimaraes, et al., "Role of 5-HT in Stress, Anxiety and Depression," *Pharmacology and Biochemical Behavior* 54 (1996): 129–141.

G. Curzon, "Effects of Food Intake on Brain Transmitter Amine Precursors and Amine Synthesis," M. Sandler and T. Silvertone, eds., *Psychopharmacology and Food,* Oxford: Oxford University Press (1985), pp. 59–70.

J. D. Fernstrom and R. J. Wurtman, "Brain Serotonin Content: Physiological Dependence on Plasma Tryptophan Levels," *Science* 174 (1971): 1023–1025.

A. Ardell, C. Garcia-Marquez, A. Armario, and E. Gelpi, "Chronic Stress Increases Serotonin and Noradrenaline in Rat Brain and Sensitizes their Response to a Further Acute Stress," *Journal of Neurochemistry* 50 (1988): 1678–1681.

C. R. Marckus, et al., "The Bovine Protein Lactalbumin Increases the Plasma Ratio of Tryptophan to the Other Large Neutral Amino Acids, and in Vulnerable Subjects Raises Brain Serotonin Activity, Reduces Cortisol Concentration, and Improves Mood under Stress," *American Journal of Clinical Nutrition* 71 (2000): 1536–1544.

R. M. Sapolsky, "Why Stress Is Bad for Your Brain," *Science* 273 (1996): 749–750.

D. T. Chalmers, S. P. Kwak, A. Mansour, et al., "Corticosteroids Regulate Brain Hippocampal 5-HT 1A Receptor mRNA Expression," *Journal of Neuroscience* 13 (1993): 914–923.

J. Herbert, "Fortnightly Review: Stress, the Brain, and Mental Illness," *British Medical Journal* 315 (1997): 530–535.

Index